はしがき

　日本人の英語は分かりにくいと言われます。確かに英語には発音しにくい音が多く存在します。私は、技術研修等を受けるために来日した外国人と話す機会があります。非英語圏から来た彼らの発音は決して上手ではありません。むしろ日本人の英語の方が聞き取りやすいことがあります。しかし、日本人と違い、話の論旨はよく伝わります。どうも発音、語彙、文法などの問題ではないようです。

　アメリカの学校では、composition（英作文）の授業でエッセイライティングを徹底的に教え込みます。ここで言うエッセイとは、日本語の随筆のように自由気ままにつづるものではありません。序文で論旨をはっきりと伝え、本文で具体的な説明を重要度（もしくは時系列）で並べて説明をし、結論で論旨を再び述べて締めくくります。極めて直線的な論旨の展開であり、形もはっきり決まっています。生徒は、伝えたい内容をこのエッセイフォーマットに当てはめて作文を書き、プレゼンテーションを行います。残念ながら、このエッセイライティングは日本の学校ではあまり取り上げていないようです。

　もちろん、普段の日常英会話は型にはめることなく自由気ままにして問題ありません。しかし、これから歯科医療に携わる学生にとって必要な英語とは何でしょうか。増加する外国人患者に対し、歯科医院までの道順を説明したり、口内炎の原因を説明したり、メタルクラウンとセラミッククラウンの違いを分かりやすく説明することではないでしょうか。必要になるのはまさしくこのエッセイライティングの発想法です。

　本テキストでは、エッセイライティングの代表的なスタイル（手順の説明、原因と結果の説明、定義づけによる説明、比較による説明、分類による説明）に歯科のテーマを当てはめて練習していきます。まず、作文でしっかりと内容を作成し、その後に英語でプレゼンテーションをして身につけます。

　従来のテキストでは音声や映像を付録のCD及びDVDで視聴する形をとりました。しかし、時代の変化とともに、CD/DVDプレーヤーを所持している学生は少数派になってしまいました。そこで、本書の音声や動画はすべてスマートホンのQRコードでアクセス出来るようになっています。自宅や学校のWi-Fi環境に合わせて視聴していただければと思います。

　最後になりますが、出版に臨んで株式会社ディーネットの井上務様、木場創自様、中岩佳代様、KAMIX株式会社の田川邦雄様、そして株式会社彩匠堂の飯垣敦様には大変お世話になりました。この場をお借りして、著者一同を代表して御礼申し上げます。

2019年4月

著者代表　藤田淳一

QRコードシリーズ
動画でわかる歯科英語―16レッスンで鍛える表現力

はしがき

目　次

本書の使い方……………………………………………………………………………………………… 3

Lesson 0.　What is an outline?　アウトラインとは?………………………………………………… 6

Ⅰ. Process　プロセスの説明……………………………………………………………………………10
　Lesson 1.　How to go from the station to the dental clinic　駅から歯科医院までの道順……12
　Lesson 2.　How to brush your teeth　歯磨きの仕方………………………………………………16
　Lesson 3.　How to treat cavities　虫歯の治療の仕方………………………………………………20

Ⅱ. Cause and Effect　原因及び結果の説明……………………………………………………………24
　Lesson 4.　The causes of tooth stains　歯の着色の原因……………………………………………26
　Lesson 5.　The causes of bad breath　口臭の原因…………………………………………………30
　Lesson 6.　The causes of stomatitis　口内炎の原因………………………………………………34
　Lesson 7.　The effects of poor tooth brushing　悪い歯磨きの結果………………………………38

Ⅲ. Definition　定義づけによる説明……………………………………………………………………42
　Lesson 8.　Definition of a beautiful smile　美しい笑顔とは………………………………………44
　Lesson 9.　Definition of a good dentist　良い歯科医とは…………………………………………48

Ⅳ. Comparison　比較による説明………………………………………………………………………52
　Lesson 10.　The differences between dental schools of Japan and Australia
　　　　　　　日本と豪州の歯学部の違い……………………………………………………………54
　Lesson 11.　The differences between metal crowns and ceramic crowns
　　　　　　　メタルクラウンとセラミッククラウンの違い………………………………………58
　Lesson 12.　The differences between implants and bridges
　　　　　　　インプラントとブリッジの違い………………………………………………………62
　Lesson 13.　The differences between whitening and veneers
　　　　　　　ホワイトニングとベニアの違い………………………………………………………66

Ⅴ. Classification　分類による説明………………………………………………………………………70
　Lesson 14.　Classification of clinical departments　臨床科の分類………………………………72
　Lesson 15.　Angle's classification of occlusion　アングルの咬合の分類…………………………76
　Lesson 16.　Classification of tooth decay　う蝕の分類……………………………………………80

Outline for presentation 1 〜 16 ………………………………………………………………………85

本書の使い方

本書は、「プロセス」、「原因及び結果」、「定義づけ」、「比較」、「分類」の5つのセクションに分かれており、それぞれの特性を知るための解説と練習問題が付いています。また、各セクションには2～4のレッスンが用意されています。

レッスン0でアウトラインについて学んだら、第1セクションの解説・問題へと進んでください。

例えば、左図は第2セクションに当たる「原因及び結果」のページとなっており、上の解説ページでは、英語で原因と結果を説明する際に注意すべきことが、歯科の現場でどのように必要になるかといった具体例を交えて書かれています。

次に、英語で原因と結果を説明する際によく使う単語・フレーズの練習をします。単語・フレーズをよりスムーズに使いこなせるように、実際に英作もしてみましょう。

Lesson 4
The causes of tooth stains

Lesson 4. 歯の着色の原因
The causes of tooth stains

Message from Dr. Andy

By having my patients understand the causes, it is possible to prevent, or at least decrease the occurrence of tooth stains. It is OK to go right ahead and enjoy food and drinks. Just be sure to follow up with immediate care.

STEP 1　必要な単語の確認

次の語を日本語に直しなさい。

1. stains
2. embarrassing
3. smoking
4. tar
5. nicotine
6. tobacco
7. discolor
8. pigment
9. tannin
10. dead tooth
11. discoloration
12. necrosis
13. pulp
14. self care
15. professional care

「原因及び結果」が英語でどのように表現されているかを理解したら、レッスンに進んでください。

まずは Dr. Andy からのメッセージを読んで、そのレッスン内容が歯科医の現場でどのような重要性を持つのかを確認しましょう。

次に STEP 1 で、最終的にエッセイとプレゼンテーションをする際に必要となる単語・フレーズの練習をしましょう。

Lesson 4
The causes of tooth stains

STEP 2　英語で書いてみよう！

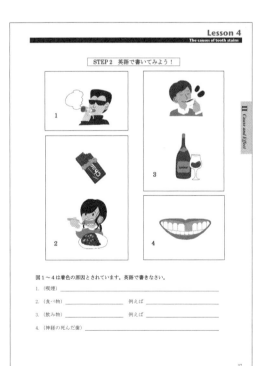

図1～4は着色の原因とされています。英語で書きなさい。

1. （喫煙）_____
2. （食べ物）_____　例えば _____
3. （飲み物）_____　例えば _____
4. （神経の死んだ歯）_____

STEP 2 は主にイラストなどを見て、それを英語にする練習パートとなっています。ここで作成したフレーズや英文を次のアウトライン作成時に使用します。

例えば、レッスン4は着色の主な原因が4つ挙げられていますので、それら4つを、具体例を交えて英語に直す作業となります。

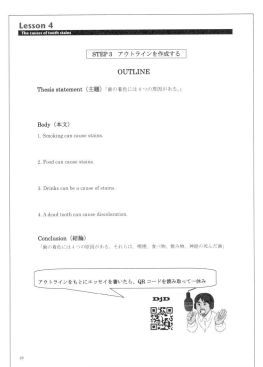

STEP 3 では前の STEP で作成したフレーズや英文を使ってアウトラインを作成します。これを元にエッセイを書いたりプレゼンテーションを行ったりすることができます。

Thesis statement（主題）でこれから自分が何を伝えるのかを明確に提示します。そして、body（本文）は前の STEP のフレーズ等を用いながら、主題の具体的な内容を書きます。最後に conclusion（結論）で、何を伝えたかったのかを再確認すると同時に、内容をまとめます。

アウトラインを元にエッセイが書けたら、DjD ロゴの下にある QR コードを読み取り、動画を見て一休みしてください。

STEP 4 は作成したエッセイをプレゼンテーションするパートになっています。まずは、モデルエッセイを何度もシャドーイングしてみてください。
次に、エッセイ内容が歯科の現場でどのように活用されているのかが動画で紹介されていますので、QR コードを読み取って見てみましょう。
最後に作成したアウトラインを見ながらでもいいので、モデルエッセイの箇所をプレゼンテーションしてみましょう。

さらに練習したい人のために応用編も用意しましたので、挑戦してみてください！

QR コード読み取り環境がない場合
以下の URL にテキスト内すべての動画があります。（パスワード：8020）
https://vimeo.com/album/5798449

Lesson. 0　アウトラインとは？
What is an outline?

私たちは普通、スピーチやプレゼンをする際に自分の言いたいことをまず箇条書きにしてから原稿をまとめたり、練習したりする。ちょっとした書き物をする時も、事前にメモを作成してこれから書く内容を自分で確認する。

この箇条書きやメモは一種の**アウトライン**と言える。
アウトラインとは自分が表現したいことの**輪郭、概略、骨組み**である。

日本語で何かを表現する際、私たちはたいてい自分が一番言いたいことを最後に述べたり、書いたりする。しかし、英語で何かを表現する場合、自分が一番言いたいことを**最初に**持ってくることが普通である。

そのため最初に自分が一番言いたいことを表す **thesis statement**（**主題文**）を書く。

例えば、AIの進化に反対の立場の場合。
Thesis statement は「わたしは AI の進化に反対だ。なぜなら、AI の進化は手放しで喜べないし、むしろ危険だからだ。」が相応しいだろう。

次になぜそのように言えるのか？といった疑問に対して具体例などを提示しながら答える必要がある。それが **body**（**本文**）となる。

例えば、以下の三つの危険性が挙げられる。
1．AI が暴走する危険性
2．管理社会に陥る危険性
3．人の成長が阻害される危険性

最後に **conclusion**（結論）を書く。

Conclusion として最もシンプルなものは、「したがって、AI には以上のような危険性があるため、私は AI の進化に反対である。」となる。Conclusion の主な役割は自分が一番言いたいことの再確認である。

これらを実際アウトラインにしてみると…

OUTLINE

I. Thesis statement（主題文）

私は AI の進化に反対だ。なぜなら、AI の進化は手放しで喜べないし、むしろ危険だからだ。

II. Body（本文）

１．AI は暴走する危険性がある。
２．世の中が管理社会に陥る危険性がある。
３．人の成長が阻害される危険性がある。

III. Conclusion（結論）

したがって、AI には以上のような危険性があるため、私は AI の進化に反対である。

最後に

最もシンプルな形のアウトラインはこれで完成だが、もう少し詳しいアウトラインを作る場合、body にあるそれぞれの項目に対していくつかの付け足しをしても良い。

例えば…
1つ目に関して…AI に関する法律等がまだ十分に整備されているとはいいがたい。
2つ目に関して…AI による人の選別化が行われるのではないか。
3つ目に関して…すべて AI 任せにすると人は思考を放棄してしまうのではないか。

以上のことを踏まえて次のテーマに関して実際にアウトラインを作ってみよう。

テーマ：私の好きな（　　　　　）は（　　　　　）だ。

※括弧の中は自由に埋めること。

STEP 1　必要な単語の確認

次の語を日本語に直しなさい。

1. first　（　　　　　　）　　　　2. second　（　　　　　　　）

3. third　（　　　　　　）　　　　4. finally　（　　　　　　　）

5. for example　（　　　　　　　）　　　6. for instance　（　　　　　　　）

7. in conclusion　（　　　　　　　）　　　8. therefore　（　　　　　　　）

9. favorite　（　　　　　　）　　　10. reason　（　　　　　　　）

11. because　（　　　　　　）　　　12. there is [are] ~　（　　　　　　　）

STEP 2　主題文を英作する

Thesis statement（主題文）：私の好きな（　　　　　）は（　　　　　）だ。
　　→　英語にすると…（　　　　　　　　　　　　　　　　　　　　　）.

STEP 3　アウトラインを作成する

OUTLINE

I. Thesis statement（主題文）

II. Body（本文）

理由を 3 つ書いてみよう。

1. (　　　　　　　　　　　　　　　　　　　　　　　　　　　　　　　　　)

2. (　　　　　　　　　　　　　　　　　　　　　　　　　　　　　　　　　)

3. (　　　　　　　　　　　　　　　　　　　　　　　　　　　　　　　　　)

III. Conclusion（結論）

アウトラインをもとにエッセイを書いたら、QR コードを読み取って一休み

全ての動画のパスワード：8020

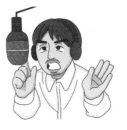

STEP 4　英語で言ってみよう！

最後にアウトラインを見ながらでもいいので、英語で言ってみよう。

I. Process ―過程を説明してみよう！
（Lesson 1 ~ 3）

Process は、作業や行為の過程を説明する方法である。普段の生活では道案内や料理の作り方を説明するときに使う。歯科医院を訪れる外国人患者に対しては次の3つの用途が考えられる。

1．　初めて来院する時の道順の説明。
2．　口腔ケアの仕方やお薬の飲み方などの説明。
3．　治療方法の説明。

英語で process の説明をするときは基本的に命令文「〜しなさい」を用いる。ただし、必要に応じて please をつけて表現を和らげるとよい。治療方法の説明の場合には、命令文の前に "I will…," や "I am going to…" をつける。それにより「〜します」というニュアンスに変わる。

Process の説明は時間の流れに沿って行う。そのため順序を示す表現を使う必要がある。日本語では「最初に」、「次に」、「最後に」を使うが、同じように英語では "first," "next," "finally" を使う。それにより、単調になりがちが説明にメリハリがついて分かりやすくなる。

例文
「歯ブラシに歯磨きをつけなさい」
Put some toothpaste on the toothbrush.
「まず真っ直ぐ進んで下さい。次に信号で右に曲がってください。」
First, go straight. Next, turn right at the traffic light.
「まず傷を消毒します。次に絆創膏をはります。」
First, I will disinfect the cut. Next, I am going to put a band aid on it.

STEP 1　必要な単語の確認

次の語を英語に直しなさい。括弧が与えられている場合は、そのアルファベットから始めること。

1．まず　　　　　　　2．次に　　　　　　　3．2番目に

4．3番目に　　　　　5．それから (t)　　　　6．そして (a)

7．最後に (f)　　　　8．最後に (l)　　　　　9．結論として (2語で)

STEP 2　英語で書いてみよう！

1．まず、バス停まで歩きます。

2．次にバスに乗って、そして京都駅で降ります。

3．3番目に、京都駅で電車に乗ります。

4．それから、大阪駅で地下鉄に乗り換えます。

5．最後に、難波駅で降りてください。

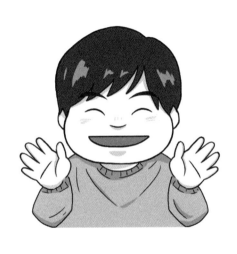

Lesson 1
How to go from the station to the dental clinic

Lesson 1. 駅から歯科医院までの道順

How to go from the station to the dental clinic

Message from Dr. Andy

When a new patient calls for directions to my clinic, I ask about their condition such as pain or detachment of prosthesis. In this way, it is possible to get everything ready before their arrival.

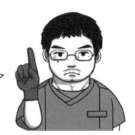

STEP 1　必要なフレーズの確認

次の各空欄を埋めなさい。

真っ直ぐ進む　→	50 メートルほど進む
Go _____	Go _____
右に曲がる　→	一つ目の交差点で右に曲がる
Turn _____	Turn _____
通り過ぎる　→	スーパーの前を通り過ぎる
Go _____	Go _____
向かって左側に医院がある	正面に医院が見えます
The clinic _____	You will find _____

Lesson 1
How to go from the station to the dental clinic

STEP 2　英語で書いてみよう！

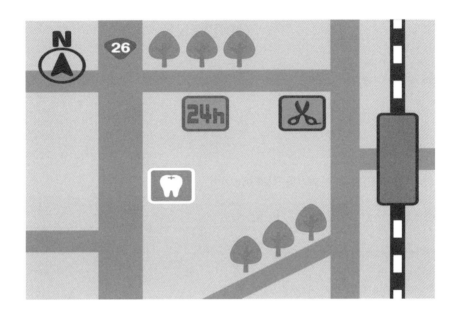

地図上の1～8で必要な命令文を英作しなさい。

1. Go out _____

2. Turn _____

3. Turn _____

4. Go _____

5. Go _____

6. Turn _____

7. Walk _____

8. The clinic is _____

Lesson 1
How to go from the station to the dental clinic

STEP 3　アウトラインを作成する

OUTLINE

Thesis statement（主題）「駅から歯科医院までの道順を説明します。約 5 分かかります。」

Body（本文）

1. Go out from the west exit of the station.

2. Turn right and walk along the street.

3. Turn left at the beauty parlor.

4. Go straight along the street.

5. Go past the convenience store.

6. Turn left at Route 26.

7. Walk straight for about 1 minute.

8. The clinic is on the left side.

Conclusion（結論）　「このようにして歯科医院に行きます。道に迷ったら遠慮なく電話してください。」

アウトラインをもとにエッセイを書いたら、QR コードを読み取って一休み

全ての動画のパスワード：8020

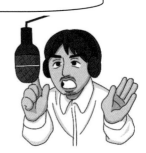

Lesson 1

How to go from the station to the dental clinic

STEP 4　英語で言ってみよう！

1．モデルエッセイでシャドーイングをしなさい。
2．現場での使われ方をDialogで確認しよう。

Dialog

Patient: Hello? Is this Andy Dental Clinic?

Andy: Yes. Dr. Andy speaking.

Patient: I am trying to find your clinic but I seem to be lost.

Andy: Where are you now?

Patient: I am at the station.

Andy: OK, here are the directions.

モデルエッセイ：**How to go from the station to the dental clinic**

(at the clinic entrance)

Andy: So you've made it.

Patient: I sure have. Your directions were on the money.

Andy: Shall we start?

Patient: OK

Andy: Change to these slippers here...This way please.

Try this in English.　応用編

How to go from my house to the university　家から大学までの道順

How to make curry and rice　カレーライスの作り方

Lesson 2. 歯磨きの仕方

How to brush your teeth

Message from Dr. Andy

Improper brushing may cause damage. In many cases, people just grip the toothbrush and apply unnecessary force to their teeth and gums. That is why I make sure my patients know how to brush properly.

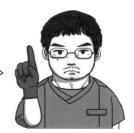

STEP 1　必要な単語の確認

次の語を日本語に直しなさい。

1. brush
2. bristles
3. apply

4. tooth surface
5. 90 degree angle
6. short strokes

7. 45 degree angle
8. outer surface
9. inner surface

10. chewing surface
11. vertically

Lesson 2
How to brush your teeth

STEP 2　英語で書いてみよう！

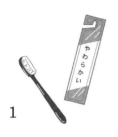
1

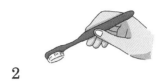
2

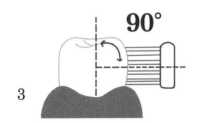
3

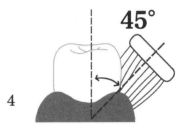
4

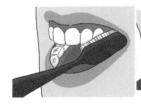
5

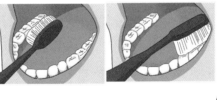

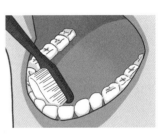
6

図1～6で必要な命令文を英作しなさい。

1. Choose _____

2. Hold _____

3. Apply _____ and brush with short strokes.

4. Apply _____ and brush with short strokes.

5. Brush _____

6. Tilt _____

Lesson 2
How to brush your teeth

> STEP 3　アウトラインを作成する

OUTLINE

Thesis statement（主題）「歯磨きの仕方を教えます。6つの手順があります。」

Body（本文）

1. Choose a toothbrush with soft bristles.

2. Hold the toothbrush with a pen grip.

3. Apply the toothbrush to the tooth surface at a 90-degree angle and brush with short strokes.

4. Apply the toothbrush to the gums at a 45-degree angle and brush with short strokes.

5. Brush the outer, inner, and chewing surfaces of the teeth.

6. Tilt the brush vertically for the inside of the front teeth.

Conclusion（結論）「このようにして歯を磨きます。」

アウトラインをもとにエッセイを書いたら、QRコードを読み取って一休み

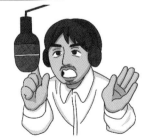

Lesson 2
How to brush your teeth

STEP 4　英語で言ってみよう！

1．モデルエッセイでシャドーイングをしなさい。
2．現場での使われ方をDialogで確認しよう。

Dialog

（染め出し中）

Andy: Hold this mirror please.
Patient: (Looking at the mirror) Oh my!
Andy: The blue parts show the plaque you had missed.
Patient: I thought I brushed my teeth thoroughly.
Andy: OK, I will tell you how to brush your teeth.
　　　　Please rinse out your mouth.

モデルエッセイ： How to brush your teeth

Andy: (Showing him the mirror) So, how does it look now?
Patient: Oh! What a difference.
Andy: You are a quick learner.
Patient: I am going to stop watching TV and focus on brushing my teeth.
Andy: That's the spirit!

Try this in English　応用編

How to floss.　フロスの仕方
How to make your favorite dish.　好きな料理の作り方
How to improve your English skills.　英語の上達方法

Lesson 3
How to treat cavities

Lesson 3. 虫歯の治療の仕方

How to treat cavities

Message from Dr. Andy

The patient should not experience any pain during the treatment. It is also important to completely remove the cause of the cavity, the decayed parts of the tooth. In the end, I make sure the filling is firmly in place.

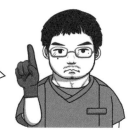

STEP 1　必要なフレーズの確認

次の語を日本語に直しなさい。

1. cavity

2. apply

3. local anesthetic

4. check

5. anesthetic

6. take effect

7. drill away

8. decay

9. fill

10. composite resin

11. shine

12. harden

13. polish

Lesson 3
How to treat cavities

STEP 2　英語で書いてみよう

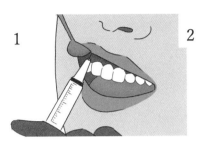
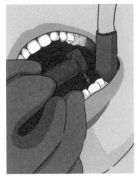
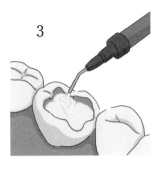
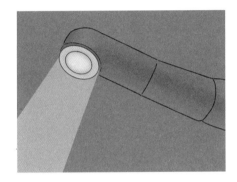
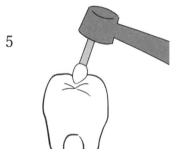

図1～5で必要な命令文を英作しなさい。

1. _____

2. _____

3. _____

4. _____

5. _____

Lesson 3
How to treat cavities

STEP 3　アウトラインを作成する

OUTLINE

Thesis statement（主題）「虫歯の治療には5つの手順がある。」

Body（本文）

1. Apply local anesthetic to the gums.

2. Drill away the decayed parts.

3. Fill with composite resin.

4. Shine light on the resin to harden.

5. Polish the surface.

Conclusion（結論）「このようにして虫歯の治療をします。」

アウトラインをもとにエッセイを書いたら、QRコードを読み取って一休み

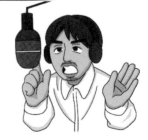

Lesson 3
How to treat cavities

> STEP 4　英語で言ってみよう！

1．モデルエッセイでシャドーイングをしなさい。
2．現場での使われ方を Dialog で確認しよう。

Dialog

(looking into the patient's mouth)

Andy: Hmm. Seems like you have a cavity.

Patient: Strange. I don't feel any pain at all.

Andy: It is still in the beginning stage.

Patient: What should I do?

Andy: I recommend treatment before it starts hurting.

Patient: How are you going to do it?

モデルエッセイ： **How to treat cavities**

Andy: Run your tongue along the edges.

Patient: Yes.

Andy: Do you feel any bumps or edges?

Patient: No I don't. It is very smooth.

Andy: Okay. We are finished.

Patient: When can I start eating?

Andy: Maybe you should wait about 1 hour.

Try this in English　応用編　　1と3に関しては具体例をつけてプレゼンテーションしなさい。

How to prevent cavities

Outline: 1. Be careful about your diet.

　　　　 2. Be sure to visit your dentist for regular checkups.

　　　　 3. Be sure to conduct daily oral care.

II. Cause & Effect—原因と結果を説明してみよう！
(Lesson 4〜7)

Cause and Effect は、物事の原因もしくは結果を説明する方法である。人を納得（説得）させるには、原因および結果を分かりやすく説明する必要がある。歯科医院を訪れる外国人患者に対しては次の3つの用途が考えられる。

1．歯科疾患の説明。（複数の原因が一つの結果）
2．矯正やインプラント治療で何が変わるか。（一つの原因が複数の結果）
3．いい加減な口腔ケアへの注意喚起。（一つの原因が複数の結果）

上記1の場合は説明の最初に "I will explain the causes of…"「これから〇〇の原因を説明します、、、」と切り出す。2と3の場合は "I am going to explain the effects of…"「これから〇〇の結果を説明します、、、」と始める。これから話す内容が causes（原因）の説明か effects（結果）の説明か最初にはっきり述べる必要がある。

続く本文ではそれぞれの原因及び結果を重要度（一番大事と思われる内容を最後に）の順番で説明する。内容によっては、前章の Process と同じく時間順で説明をする。例えばいい加減な口腔ケア（原因）がどのような結果を招くかについて話す場合、症状が進行していく順で説明をすることもできる。（poor care→bacteria accumulates→formation of plaque→formation of periodontal pockets→periodontal disease）

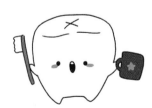

STEP 1　必要な単語の確認

次の語を英語に直しなさい。括弧が与えられている場合は、そのアルファベットから始めること。

結果を表す単語やフレーズ：

1．〜という結果になる（r、2語で）　　2．結果として（a、3語で）

3．したがって（t）　　　　　　　　　4．したがって（t）

5．したがって（c）　　　　　　　　　6．したがって（h）

7．したがって（s）　　　　　　　　　8．したがって（t）

原因を表す単語やフレーズ：

1．〜というのは（f）　　　　　　　　2．なぜなら（b）

3．なぜなら（s）　　　　　　　　　　4．なぜなら（a）

5．〜が原因で（d, 2語で）　　　　　　6．〜が原因で（o, 3語で）

7．〜によって（b）

STEP 2　英語で書いてみよう！

1．激しい歯磨きは歯茎のダメージにつながりうる。

2．私は食べ過ぎた。その結果、私のジーンズはきつい。

3．口臭はニンニクの入った食べ物が多すぎることが原因だ。

4．歯垢は砂糖をエサとする細菌によって形成される。

Lesson 4. 歯の着色の原因

The causes of tooth stains

Message from Dr. Andy

By having my patients understand the causes, it is possible to prevent, or at least decrease the occurrence of tooth stains. It is OK to go right ahead and enjoy food and drinks. Just be sure to follow up with immediate care.

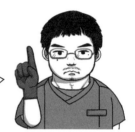

STEP 1　必要な単語の確認

次の語を日本語に直しなさい。

1. stains
2. embarrassing
3. smoking

4. tar
5. nicotine
6. tobacco

7. discolor
8. pigment
9. tannin

10. dead tooth
11. discoloration
12. necrosis

13. pulp
14. self care
15. professional care

Lesson 4
The causes of tooth stains

STEP 2　英語で書いてみよう！

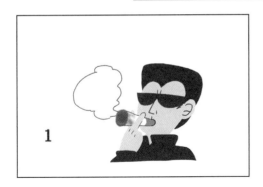

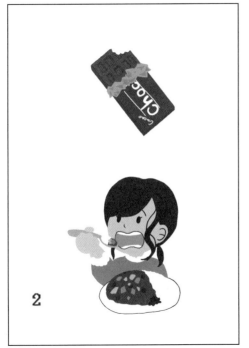

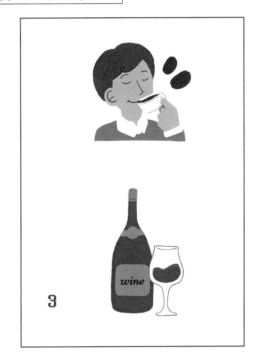

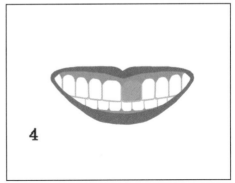

図1〜4は着色の原因とされています。英語で書きなさい。

1. （喫煙）_____

2. （食べ物）_____　例えば _____

3. （飲み物）_____　例えば _____

4. （神経の死んだ歯）_____

Lesson 4
The causes of tooth stains

STEP 3　アウトラインを作成する

OUTLINE

Thesis statement（主題）「歯の着色には4つの原因がある。」

Body（本文）

1. Smoking can cause stains.

2. Food can cause stains.

3. Drinks can be a cause of stains.

4. A dead tooth can cause discoloration.

Conclusion（結論）
　「歯の着色には4つの原因がある。それらは、喫煙、食べ物、飲み物、神経の死んだ歯」

アウトラインをもとにエッセイを書いたら、QRコードを読み取って一休み

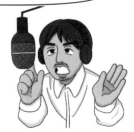

Lesson 4
The causes of tooth stains

STEP 4　英語で言ってみよう！

1．モデルエッセイでシャドーイングをしなさい。
2．現場での使われ方を Dialog で確認しよう。

Dialog

Patient: Dr. Andy, I've made it to the final job interview.
Andy: That is good news! But I also have some bad news too.
Patient: What?
Andy: You have quite a lot of stains on your teeth.
Patient: (looking into the mirror) Oh my!

モデルエッセイ：　The causes of tooth stains

(following the treatment)
Patient: (looking into the mirror) Wow! What a difference.
Andy: So, now you are ready for the interview.
Patient: Do you have any tips?
Andy: Be sure to smile and show them your beautiful teeth.

Try this in English 応用編　アウトラインを作成して英語でプレゼンしよう。
タイトル　I am healthy / not healthy

1．_____

2．_____

3．_____

注：必ず具体例（for example）をつけること。

Lesson 5

Lesson 5. 口臭の原因

The causes of bad breath

Message from Dr. Andy

There are studies that indicate Japanese people pay less attention towards their own breath. When traveling abroad or meeting with a foreign person, be especially careful about your breath.

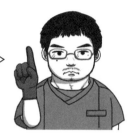

STEP 1　必要な単語の確認

次の語を日本語に直しなさい。

1. displeasing

2. bad breath

3. strong smelling

4. smell foul

5. poor

6. oral care

7. insufficient

8. lack of

9. flossing

10. influence

11. oral disease

12. periodontitis

13. proper

14. knowledge

15. regular checkups

16. prevent

Lesson 5
The causes of bad breath

STEP 2　英語で書いてみよう！

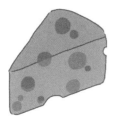
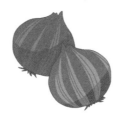
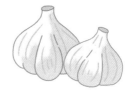

Cause 1　（食べ物、食習慣）_____

　　　For example, _____

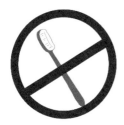
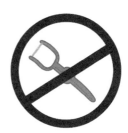

Cause 2　（悪い口腔衛生習慣）_____

　　　For example, _____

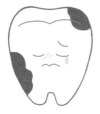
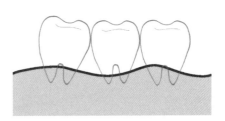

Cause 3　（口腔内の病気）_____

　　　For example, _____

Lesson 5
The causes of bad breath

STEP 3　アウトラインを作成する

OUTLINE

Thesis statement（主題）「口臭には3つの原因がある。」

Body（本文）（3つの原因を英語で書きなさい。）

1. 食べ物が口臭の原因になることがある。

2. 悪い口腔衛生習慣が口臭の原因になりうる。

3. 口臭は口腔内の病気の症状かもしれない。

Conclusion（結論）「口臭は食べ物、ケア不足、口腔内の病気によって引き起こされる。」

アウトラインをもとにエッセイを書いたら、QRコードを読み取って一休み

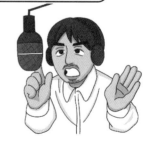

QRコードシリーズ
動画でわかる歯科英語
― 16レッスンで鍛える表現力 ―
解答集

著　　　者	藤田淳一／岡　隼人／安東大器
	岡村友玄／吉川美弘
発　行　者	杉田宗詞
発　行　所	図書出版 浪速社
	〒540-0037　大阪市中央区内平野町２−２−７−502
	TEL 06（6942）5032　FAX 06（6943）1346
印刷・製本	株式会社ディーネット

―禁無断転載―

2019年 © 藤田淳一／岡　隼人／安東大器／岡村友玄／吉川美弘

乱丁落丁はお取り替えいたします
ISBN978-4-88854-521-1

remain. In conclusion, tooth decay can be divided into five stages depending on progression of decay.
（モデルエッセイ和訳）
　う蝕は進行の度合いにより5つのステージに分類することができる。最初のステージはC0です。このステージではう蝕が始まりかけています。次のステージはC1です。このステージではエナメル質がう蝕にかかっています。次のステージはC2です。このステージではう蝕が象牙質まで進行しています。次のステージはC3です。このステージでは歯髄が侵されています。次のステージはC4です。このステージでは、歯の歯根のみが残っています。従いまして、う蝕は進行の度合いにより5つのステージに分けることができる。

患者：と言うことは虫歯が何本かあるということなの？
アンディー先生：残念ながら、はい。
患者：あらまあ！
アンディー先生：ご心配なく。まだ初期の段階なので、これ以上の進行を止めることができます。
患者：よかった。早速お願いね！

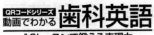

12. depend on ～によって

Step 2

分類の基準：progression

う蝕になりかけている：The decay is about to start.

エナメル質がう蝕にかかっている：The enamel is decayed.

う蝕は象牙質に進んでいる：The decay has advanced to the dentin.

歯髄が侵されている：The pulp has been affected.

歯根のみが残っている：Only the roots of the tooth remain.

Step 3

Thesis statement:

　Tooth decay can be classified into five stages according to progression.

Body:

1. In this stage, the decay is about to start.
2. In this stage, the enamel is decayed.
3. In this stage, the decay has advanced to the dentin.
4. In this stage, the pulp has been affected
5. In this stage, only the roots of the tooth remain.

Conclusion:

　Tooth decay can be classified into five stages depending on progression of decay.

Step 4

Dialog（和訳）

　（アンディー先生はサリーの診察を行っている。彼の助手が表に詳細を書きとっている。）

患者：アンディー先生、私は日本語は分からないけど、「c なんとか」って言っているのが何度も聞こえるような気がするわ。

アンディー先生：ちょうど今、結果を説明するところでした。

患者：あれはどういう意味なの？

モデルエッセイ

　Tooth decay can be classified into five stages according to progression. The first stage is C0. In this stage, the decay is about to start. The second stage is C1. In this stage, the enamel is decayed. The third stage is C2. In this stage, the decay has advanced to the dentin. The fourth stage is C3. In this stage, the pulp has been affected. The fifth stage is C4. In this stage, only the roots of the teeth

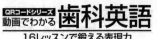

Occlusion can be divided into three classes according to the position of the jaws and teeth.

Step 4
Dialog（和訳）
患者：特定の言葉が発音しづらいことがあります。
アンディー先生：おそらく噛み合わせが原因だと思います。
患者：ずっと自分の噛み合わせは普通だと思っていましたが。
アンディー先生：見てみましょう…「イー」してください。
患者：それで、どういった具合ですか。

モデルエッセイ

　Occlusion can be classified into three types according to relation between teeth and jaws. The first classification is class I. The relationship between teeth and jaws is normal in this group. The second classification is class II or overbite. The upper front teeth and jaw project further forward than the lower teeth and jaw. The third classification is class III or underbite. In this case, the lower teeth and jaw project further forward than the upper teeth and jaws. So, occlusion can be classified into three classes according to the position of the teeth and jaws.

（モデルエッセイ和訳）
　咬合は歯と顎の関係において3つに分類することができます。最初の分類はクラス1です。このグループでは歯と顎の関係は普通です。次の分類はクラス2もしくは過蓋咬合と呼ばれます。上顎の前歯が下の歯と顎よりさらに前突しています。次の分類はクラス3もしくは反対咬合と呼ばれます。この場合は、下顎の歯と顎が上の歯と顎よりさらに前突しています。従いまして、咬合は歯と顎の位置に基づいて3つのクラスに分類することができる。

アンディー先生：わずかですが、前歯が出ていますね。対処できますよ。
患者：どうするんですか？
アンディー先生：矯正治療です。
患者：えぇ！あの金属のわっかですか？
アンディー先生：それはもう過去の話です。（サンプルを彼に見せる）

Lesson 16. う蝕の分類

Step 1
1. tooth decay う蝕　2. according to 〜によって　3. progression 進具合
4. be about to〜し始める　5. enamel エナメル質　6. advance to〜へ進む　7. pulp 歯髄
8. affected 侵される 9. roots 歯根 10. remain 残存する　11. be divided into〜に分ける

orthodontics according to treatment.

（モデルエッセイ和訳）
　歯科における臨床は、治療内容別に4つのグループに分類することができます。最初のグループは補綴です。治療はインプラント、ブリッジ、義歯などの補綴物の設置を含みます。次のグループは保存です。治療は充填、根管治療、歯周処置を含みます。次のグループは口腔外科です。抜歯などの処置が含まれます。次のグループは、矯正歯科です。治療には歯列の矯正が含まれています。従いまして、歯科における臨床は治療内容により補綴、保存、口腔外科そして矯正歯科に分類することができる。

患者：なるほど。と言うことは、私は口腔外科に紹介されるんですね。
アンディー先生：その通りです。
患者：矯正はいつから再開できますか？
アンディー先生：だいたい1か月から2か月後でしょう。

Lesson 15. アングルの咬合の分類

Step 1

1. occlusion 咬合　2. relation 関係　3. classification 分類　4. overbite オーバーバイト
5. upper teeth 上顎の歯　6. project 突き出る　7. further forward より前方
8. lower teeth 下顎の歯　9. underbite アンダーバイト

Step 2

分類の基準：Relation between teeth and jaws

Class I: normal

Class II: overbite

Class III: underbite

Step 3

Thesis statement:
　Occlusion can be classified into three types according to relation between teeth and jaws.

Body:

1. The relationship between teeth and jaws is normal in this group.
2. The upper front teeth and jaw project further forward than the lower teeth and jaw.
3. The lower teeth and jaw project further forward than the upper teeth and jaw.

Conclusion:

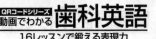

1. 補綴：prosthodontics
2. 保存修復：operative dentistry
3. 口腔外科：oral surgery
4. 矯正：orthodontics

Step 3

Thesis statement:

　Clinics in dentistry can be classified into four groups by treatment.

Body:

　1. Prosthodontics: involves placement of prosthesis such as implants, bridges or dentures.
　2. Operative dentistry: includes fillings, root canal treatment, and periodontal procedures.
　3. Oral surgery: includes such procedures as tooth extractions.
　4. Orthodontics: includes correction of tooth alignment.

Conclusion:

　Clinics in dentistry can be classified into prosthodontics, restoration, oral surgery, and orthodontics according to treatment.

Step 4

Dialog（和訳）

アンディー先生：奥歯を抜かないといけませんね。
患者：どの歯ですか？
アンディー先生：左下の奥歯です。
患者：痛いですか？
アンディー先生：ご心配なく。歯科病院をご紹介します。腕はピカイチです。
患者：歯科病院ですか！どの診療科に私は行くのですか？

モデルエッセイ

　Clinics in dentistry can be classified into four groups by treatment. The first group is prosthodontics. The treatment involves placement of prosthesis such as implants, bridges or dentures. The second group is restoration. This includes fillings, root canal treatment, and periodontal procedures. The third group is oral surgery. This includes such procedures as tooth extractions. The fourth group is orthodontics. Treatment includes correction of tooth alignment. In conclusion, clinics in dentistry can be classified into prosthodontics, restoration, oral surgery, and

アンディー先生：ホワイトニングを試されてはいかがですか？

患者：そうですね…また時間とお金がある時に、ベニアを考えてみるわ。

V. Classification—分類してみよう！（Lesson 14～16）

Step 1

1．～に分類できる（c、4語で）
　can be classified into
2．グループ
　group
3．タイプ
　type
4．～にしたがって（a、2語で）
　according to
5．分類（c）
　classification
6．段階（s）
　step
7．～にしたがって（d、2語で）
　depending on
8．～に基づいて（o、4語で）
　on the basis of
9．種類（k）
　kind

Step 2

1．血液型は4つに分類できる。
　Blood type can be classified into 4 types.
2．建物は利用法に基づいて3つに分類できる。
　Buildings can be classified into three groups on the basis of use.
3．ワインはその砂糖含有率（their sugar content）にしたがって分類できる。
　Wine can be classified according to their sugar content.

Lesson 14. 臨床科の分類

Step 1

1. clinics 臨床　2. classify 分類する　3. Prosthodontics 補綴科
4. involve / include 関係する/含む　5. placement 設置　6. prosthesis 補綴物
7. denture 義歯　8. restoration 修復　9. fillings 詰め物
10. root canal treatment 根管治療　11. procedures 処置　12. Oral surgery 口腔外科
13. tooth extraction 抜歯　14. Orthodontics 矯正科　15. correction 修正
16. tooth alignment 歯列　17. according to ～にもとづいて

Step 2

分類の基準： treatment

2. invasiveness	not invasive	invasive
3. cost	40,000 yen	100,000 yen
4. duration	a few years	5 to 10 years

Conclusion: Whitening treatment and veneer treatment have four differences.

Step 4

Dialog（和訳）

患者：今度、たくさんの人の前でプレゼンするの。
アンディー先生：ワクワクしますね。
患者：でも、ちょっと見た目で心配なことが…
アンディー先生：どこがですが？
患者：私の歯の色が…

モデルエッセイ

　　Whitening treatment and veneer treatment have four differences. First, whitening is the application of chemicals to the teeth. On the other hand, veneers are porcelain covers attached to the teeth. Second, whitening is not invasive. However, veneers are invasive. The tooth surface needs drilling. Third, whitening costs about 40,000 yen per treatment. In contrast, veneers cost 100,000 yen per tooth. Fourth, the effect of whitening lasts for a few years. However, veneers last between 5 to 10 years. In conclusion, whitening treatment and veneer treatment have four differences.

（モデルエッセイ和訳）

　　ホワイトニング治療とベニア治療には４つの違いがあります。まず、ホワイトニングでは歯に薬品を塗布します。一方で、ベニアでは歯に陶材のカバーを接着します。次に、ホワイトニングは侵襲性がありません。しかし、ベニアは侵襲性があります。歯の表面を削る必要があります。次に、ホワイトニングは一回の治療に４万円ほどかかります。それに対して、ベニアは一本あたり10万円かかります。次に、ホワイトニングの効果は数年間続きます。一方、ベニアは５〜10年持ちます。従って、ホワイトニング治療とベニア治療には４つの違いがあります。

アンディー先生：プレゼンはいつですか？
患者：来週です。

（モデルエッセイ和訳）
　インプラントとブリッジには4つの違いがあります。まず、インプラントは隣接する歯に負荷をかけません。それに対して、ブリッジは隣接する歯に負荷をかけます。多少、削る必要があります。次に、インプラントの維持にはセルフケアとプロケアの両方が必要です。しかし、ブリッジの維持はセルフケアで行います。次に、インプラント治療には時間がかかります。一方で、ブリッジは短時間ですみます。次に、インプラントの費用は高いです。それに対して、ブリッジの費用は高くありません。従って、インプラントとブリッジには4つの違いがあります。

患者：さて、これは本当に難しい選択だ。
ムッティ先生：経済的に余裕があるのでしたら、インプラントの方をおすすめします。
患者：そうですね、他の歯を削られるのは嫌ですし。
ムッティ先生：奥の私のお部屋に来ていただければ、もっと詳しい説明をさせていただきます。
患者：(ﾟДﾟ)

Lesson 13. ホワイトニングとベニアの違い

Step 1
1. whitening ホワイトニング　2. veneer ベニア　3. application 塗布　4. chemicals 薬品
5. porcelain 陶材　6. attach 接着　7. invasive 侵襲性がある　8. drilling 削ること
9. cost かかる　10. per treatment 一回の治療につき　11. in contrast それに対して
12. effect　効果

Step 2
ホワイトニング：
1. 方法：chemicals　2. 侵襲性：not invasive　3. コスト：40,000 yen　4. 耐久年数：a few years
ベニア：
1. 方法：attachment　2. 侵襲性：invasive　3. コスト：100,000 yen　4. 耐久年数：5 to 10 years

Step 3
Thesis statement: Whitening treatment and veneer treatment have four differences.

Body:

対比の項目↓	whitening	veneer
1. method	chemicals	attachment

Step 3

Thesis statement:

　Implants and bridges have four differences.

Body:

対比の項目↓	implants	bridges
1. strain on nearby teeth	no strain	strain
2. maintenance	professional care and self-care	self-care
3. time	long	short
4. cost	expensive	inexpensive

Conclusion:

　Implants and bridges have four differences.

Step 4

Dialog（和訳）

ムッティ先生：本当にひどい事故でしたね。

患者：ええ。生きていることが信じがたいほどです。

ムッティ先生：これから失くされた歯があった隙間をどうにかしないといけません。

患者：どんな治療が可能ですか？

ムッティ先生：ブリッジかインプラントが可能ですね。

患者：違いは何ですか？

モデルエッセイ

　Implants and bridges have four differences. First, implants do not put strain on nearby teeth. In contrast, bridges place strain on nearby teeth. Some drilling is necessary. Second, the maintenance of implants require both self-care and professional care. However, the maintenance of bridges is self-care. Third, time is necessary for implant treatment while bridges take a short time. Fourth, the cost of implants is expensive whereas the cost of bridges is not. In conclusion, implants and bridges have four differences.

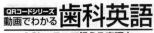

アンディー先生：金属かセラミックかで選べますよ。

患者：違いは何？

モデルエッセイ

　Metal crowns and ceramic crowns have four differences. First, metal crowns are insured. However, ceramic crowns are not insured. Second, metal crowns have a metallic appearance. On the other hand, ceramic crowns have a natural appearance. Third, metal crowns are durable whereas ceramic crowns may crack. Finally, metal crowns may cause allergy though ceramic crowns do not. So, metal crowns and ceramic crowns have four differences.

（モデルエッセイ和訳）

　メタルクラウンとセラミッククラウンの間には４つの違いがあります。まずメタルクラウンには保険が適用されます。しかし、セラミッククラウンには適用されません。次に、メタルクラウンの外見は金属です。一方でセラミッククラウンの外見は自然です。次に、メタルクラウンは耐久性があります。それに対し、セラミッククラウンは欠けることがあります。次に、メタルクラウンはアレルギーを引き起こす可能性があります。しかし、セラミッククラウンはありません。従って、メタルクラウンとセラミッククラウンには４つの違いがあります。

患者：金属にしようかしら。

アンディー先生：それはいい選択です。奥歯に被せるので、頑丈な方がいいですし。

患者：目立たなければいいけど、、、

アンディー先生：あくびをする時は手でお口を隠すように。

Lesson 12. インプラントとブリッジの違い

Step 1

1. implants インプラント　2. bridge ブリッジ　3. strain 負荷　4. nearby 隣接する

5. drilling 削ること　6. maintenance 維持　7. require 必要とする　8. self-care セルフケア

9. professional care プロケア　10. long time 長時間　11. short time 短時間

Step 2

インプラント：

1. 隣接歯への負荷：no strain　2. メンテナンス：self-care and professional care　3. 時間：long time　4. 費用：expensive

ブリッジ：

1. 隣接歯への負荷：strain　2. メンテナンス：self-care　3. 時間：short time　4. 費用：inexpensive

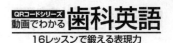

1. insured 保険適用 2. not insured 保険適用外 3. metallic 金属のような
4. appearance 外見 5. natural 自然な 6. durable 耐久性がある 7. crack 欠ける
8. allergy アレルギー

Step 2

メタルクラウン
1. 保険適用：insured 2. 見た目：metallic 3. 強度：durable 4. アレルギー反応：metal allergy
セラミッククラウン
1. 保険適用：not insured 2. 見た目：natural 3. 強度：crack 4. アレルギー反応：no allergy

Step 3

Thesis statement:

　Metal crowns and ceramic crowns have four differences.

Body:

対比の項目↓	**metal crown**	**ceramic crown**
1. 保険適用 insurance	insured	not insured
2. 見た目 appearance	metallic	natural
3. 強度 strength	durable	might crack
4. アレルギー反応 allergic reaction	metal allergy	no allergy

Conclusion:

　Metal crowns and ceramic crowns have four differences.

Step 4

Dialog（和訳）

アンディー先生：クラウンを付けるための歯の準備が完了しましたよ。
患者：次は何をするの？
アンディー先生：クラウンの種類を決めなくてはなりません。
患者：どんな種類があるの？

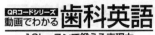

Step 4

Dialog（和訳）

アンディー：お口をゆすいでください。今日はこれでおしまいです。また来週、来てください。

患者：ありがとう。ところで、いつからここで患者を診ているの？

アンディー先生：国家試験に合格してからですね…10年前くらい前のことです。

患者：卒業した後に試験を受けないといけないの？

アンディー先生：はい、免許取得のために。

患者：シドニーにいる友達は卒業後すぐに患者を診ていたわよ。

アンディー先生：日本とオーストラリアでは制度が異なります。

モデルエッセイ

　Dental schools in Japan and Australia have four differences. First, high school graduates can apply for dental school in Japan. On the other hand, only college graduates with a BA or above can apply for dental school in Australia. Second, Japanese dental schools are six year courses while Australian dental schools are four year courses. Third, Japanese dental students start clinics from the fifth year. In contrast, Australian dental students start clinics from the second year. Finally, students must graduate and pass the national board examination to become a licensed dentist in Japan. However, students become licensed dentists upon graduation in Australia. In conclusion, there are mainly four differences between dental schools in Japan and Australia.

（モデルエッセイ和訳）

　日本とオーストラリアの歯学部には4つの違いがあります。まず、日本の歯学部は、高校卒業の資格で受験することができます。一方でオーストラリアの歯学部は4年制大学卒業の学士かそれ以上の資格を持った人が受験できます。次に、日本の歯学部は6年生であるのに対して、オーストラリアの歯学部は4年制です。次に、日本の歯学部生は5年生から臨床実習を開始します。一方でオーストラリアの歯学部生は2年目から臨床実習を始めます。次に、日本で歯科医になるためには、卒業をして国家試験に合格しなければなりません。しかし、オーストラリアでは、卒業と同時に歯科医師になります。従って、日本とオーストラリアの歯学部には主に4つの違いがあります。

患者：なるほど。どちらの国でも歯科医師になるには大変な努力が必要なのね。

アンディー先生：ええ。でも、とりわけ患者さんの笑顔を見ると、やりがいのある仕事だと感じますね。

患者：こんな風に？（微笑む）

アンディー先生：そうですね…ただ、まだ口をゆすいでいませんね。

Lesson 11. メタルクラウンとセラミッククラウンの違い

Step 1

Lesson 10. 日本と豪州の歯学部の違い

Step 1

1. dental school 歯学部　2. differences 違い　3. high school graduate 高卒
4. apply for　〜を受験する　5. college graduate 大卒　6. BA 学士
7. six year course　6年制　8. clinics 臨床実習　9. graduate 卒業する
10. national board examination 国家試験　11. licensed dentist（資格を持った）歯科医師
12. upon graduation 卒業してすぐ

Step 2

日本の歯学部
1. 受験者：high school graduate　2. 年数：6 years　3. 臨床実習開始年：5th year　4. 資格取得：national board examination

オーストラリアの歯学部
1. 受験者：college graduates　2. 年数：4 years　3. 臨床実習開始年：2nd year　4. 資格取得：graduation

Step 3

Thesis statement:
　　Dental schools in Japan and Australia have four differences.

Body:

何を比較するか　↓	Japan	Australia
1.（受験者） applicants	high school graduates	college graduates
2.（就学年数） course	6 year course	4 year course
3.（臨床実習開始年次） start of clinics	5th year	2nd year
4.（資格取得） qualification	national board exam	graduation

Conclusion:
There are mainly four differences between dental schools in Japan and Australia.

女性：よさげな歯科医師みたいだね。
男性：実は、彼のクリニックはそこの角を曲がったところにあるよ。
女性：ホント？連れて行ってくれるかしら？
男性：もちろん、いいとも。さぁ…
アンディー先生：こんにちは。サリーさんですか？さぁ、こちらへ。
男性：（状況に気づいて勘定を手に取る）

IV. Comparison—比較して説明してみよう！（Lesson 10～13）

Step 1
相違点：
1. 対照的に（i、2 語で）
   in contrast
2. 一方で（o、4 語で）
   on the other hand
3. しかしながら（h）
   however
4. 一方で（w）
   while
5. 一方で（w）
   whereas
6. しかし（b）
   but
7. しかし（y）
   yet

類似点：
1. 同様に（l）
   likewise
2. 同様に（s）
   similarly
3. さらに（a）
   also
4. 〜とおり（j、2 語で）
   just at
5. 〜と〜とともに（b）
   both

Step 2
1. リンゴは赤い。しかしながら、バナナは黄色い。
   Apples are red. However, bananas are yellow.
2. アメリカ合衆国は大きな国である一方で、日本は小さい。
   While the United States of America is a large country, Japan is small.
3. コーヒーは山で栽培される。同様に、お茶も高地で栽培される。
   Coffee is grown in the mountains. Likewise, tea is grown in highlands.
4. ロシアは中国もそうである通り大きな国だ。
   Russia is a large country just as China.

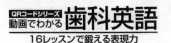

Body:
1. A good dentist has communication skills.
2. A good dentist has respect for their patients.
3. A good dentist has a firm knowledge of dentistry.
4. A good dentist has (requires) good treatment skills.

Conclusion

 A good dentist has communication skills, respect for their patients, firm knowledge, and skills in dentistry.

Step 4

Dialog（和訳）

女性：いつも同じ歯科医師に見てもらっているの？
男性：うん。定期検診を受けに行ってるよ。
女性：彼は英語が達者なの？
男性：かなり達者だよ…それだけじゃなくて、彼は…

モデルエッセイ

 A good dentist has four qualities: communication skills, respect for patients, firm knowledge, and treatment skills.

 First, a good dentist has communication skills. The skills help establish good rapport with the patient. Second, a good dentist has respect for their patients. The patient in turn will respect their dentist. Third, a good dentist has a firm knowledge of dentistry. They can answer any question or inquiry raised by the patient. Finally, a good dentist requires good treatment skills. This is necessary to help regain the oral health of the patients.

 In conclusion, a good dentist has communication skills, respect for their patients, firm knowledge, and treatment skills.

（モデルエッセイ和訳）

 良い歯科医には4つの要素があります。それは、コミュニケーション術、患者への尊敬の気持ち、しっかりとした知識そして治療の技術です。まず、良い歯科医はコミュニケーション術があります。このスキルにより患者との信頼関係を構築します。次に、良い歯科医は患者に対して尊敬の気持ちがあります。患者も自分の歯科医を尊敬するようになります。次に、良い歯科医は歯学の知識をしっかりもっています。患者からのどのような質問にも答えることができます。次に、良い歯科医には良い技術が必要です。患者のお口の健康を取り戻すのに必要です。従って、良い歯科医はコミュニケーション術、患者への尊敬、しっかりとした知識そして治療の技術を持ち合わせています。

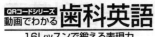

　The first factor is good teeth alignment. Orthodontic treatment will help to fix crooked teeth and irregular teeth. The second factor is teeth color. Whitening treatment can help treat discolored teeth. The third factor is facial expression. It is necessary to convey your feelings with rich facial expressions.

　In conclusion, the three factors to get a beautiful smile are good teeth alignment, good teeth color, and rich facial expressions. For a beautiful smile, visit your dentist today.

（モデルエッセイ和訳）

　美しい笑顔は自信を与えます。良い笑顔を得るには3つの要素が必要である。それらは、歯並び、歯の色そして表情です。1つ目の要素は、良い歯並びです。矯正治療は歯並びを直してくれます。2つ目の要素は歯の色です。ホワイトニング治療は変色した歯を直してくれます。3つ目の要素は表情です。豊かな表情で気持ちを伝える必要があります。従って、美しい笑顔のための3つの要素は、よい歯並び、きれいな歯の色そして豊かな表情です。歯科医院を訪れて美しい笑顔になりましょう。

患者：美しい笑顔は私の新しい仕事にきっと役立つでしょうね。
ムッティ先生：歯のホワイトニングを試してみますか？
患者：ええ、すぐにでも。
ムッティ先生：まずはそのネクタイを外しましょうか。
患者：(ﾟДﾟ)

Lesson 9. 良い歯科医とは

Step 1

1. good 良い　2. qualities 特質　3. communication skills コミュニケーション能力
4. respect 尊敬　5. firm しっかりとした　6. skills 技術　7. establish 確立する
8. rapport 疎通　9. in turn 逆に　10. dentistry 歯学
11. question / inquiry 質問・問い合わせ　12. regain 取り戻す

Step 2

1. communication skills
2. respect for patients
3. firm knowledge
4. treatment skills

Step 3

Thesis statement:
　A good dentist has four qualities.

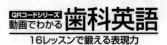

1. confidence 自信　2. factor 要素　3. teeth alignment 歯並び　4. facial expression 表情
5. orthodontic treatment 矯正治療　6. crooked teeth 悪い歯並び
7. irregular 不規則な　8. whitening treatment ホワイトニング　9. convey 伝える　10. rich 豊かな

Step 2

1. teeth alignment

具体的に：Orthodontic treatment will help fix crooked teeth and irregular bites.

2. teeth color

具体的に：Whitening treatment can help treat discolored teeth.

3. facial expressions

具体的に：Rich facial expressions will convey your feelings.

Step 3

Thesis statement:

　Three factors are necessary to get a good-looking smile.

Body:

1. The first factor is good teeth alignment.
2. The second factor is teeth color.
3. The third factor is facial expressions.

Conclusion:

　The three factors to get a beautiful smile are good teeth alignment, good teeth color, and rich facial expressions.

Step 4

Dialog（和訳）

ムッティ先生：いいネクタイをされてますね。
患者：どうも。スーツを新調したところでして。
ムッティ先生：イメチェンってやつですか？
患者：ええ、転職に合わせてね…これ以外に何かできることはないかなと思っていまして。
ムッティ先生：あなたの笑顔を変えられますよ。
患者：どうやって？

モデルエッセイ

　A beautiful smile brings confidence. Three factors are necessary to get a nice looking smile. They are teeth alignment, teeth color, and facial expression.

モデルエッセイ

　Poor tooth brushing has a negative effect on oral health. There are four negative effects to poor tooth brushing. First, poor tooth brushing can lead to tooth stains. Second, poor tooth brushing will lead to tooth decay. Plaque can build up and attack the tooth enamel. Third, poor tooth brushing can bring about gum trouble. Bacteria can build up below the gum. Fourth, as a result of tooth decay and gum trouble, tooth loss can occur. In conclusion, poor tooth brushing can lead to tooth stains, tooth decay, gum trouble, and eventually tooth loss. It is important to visit the dentist for assessment of oral health.

（モデルエッセイ和訳）

　よくない歯磨き（歯磨き不足）はお口の健康に悪影響を与えます。よくない歯磨きは4つの悪い結果をもたらします。まず、歯の着色につながるかも知れません。次に、よくない歯磨きはう蝕をもたらします。歯垢がたまって歯のエナメル質を侵すことがあります。次に、歯肉のトラブルをもたらすことがあります。歯茎の下にバクテリアが蓄積します。次に、う蝕や歯肉のトラブルの結果として、歯の喪失が起きることがあります。従って、よくない歯磨きは着色、う蝕、歯肉トラブルそしてやがて歯の喪失へとつながるかもしれません。歯科医院でお口の健康状態を診てもらうことが大切です。

患者：何てこった！ホラー映画みたいじゃないか。
アンディー先生：うちの歯科衛生士が適切な歯の磨き方を教えますよ。
患者ジ：（可愛く若い歯科助手を期待して）すぐお願いします！
アンディー先生：（奥から男が現れて）こんちは。担当をします歯科衛生士です。
患者：（ゾッとしている表情）(ﾟДﾟ)

III. Definition―定義づけて説明してみよう！（Lesson 8～9）

Step 1

1．whale　2．kitchen　3．river　4．spider　5．muscle

Step 2

1．ゾウ　An elephant is a very large grey mammal that has a long nose called a trunk.
2．10月　October is the tenth month of the year.
3．地球　The earth is the third planet from the sun.
4．バナナ　A banana is a long, curved fruit with a yellow skin.
5．歯科医師　A dentist is a person whose job is treating teeth.

Lesson 8. 美しい笑顔とは

Step 1

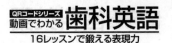

1. poor tooth brushing　よくない歯磨き　2. negative 悪い　3. oral health 口腔の健康
4. tooth stains 着色　5. tooth decay う蝕　6. plaque 歯垢　7. build up 蓄積する
8. attack 侵す　9. tooth enamel エナメル質　10. bring about もたらす
11. gum trouble 歯茎のトラブル　12. bacteria 細菌　13. as a result of 〜の結果
14. tooth loss 歯の喪失　15. occur 発生する　16. eventually やがて　17. assessment 評価

Step 2

Effect 1: tooth stains

Effect 2: tooth decay

   Plaque can build up and attack the tooth enamel.

Effect 3: gum trouble

   Bacteria can build up below the gum.

Effect 4: tooth loss

   Tooth loss occurs as a result of tooth decay and gum trouble.

Step 3

Thesis statement:

 There are four negative effects to poor tooth brushing.

Body:

1. Poor tooth brushing can lead to tooth stains.
2. Poor tooth brushing will lead to tooth decay.
3. Poor tooth brushing can bring about gum trouble.
4. As a result of tooth decay and gum trouble, tooth loss can occur.

Conclusion:

 Poor tooth brushing can lead to tooth stains, tooth decay, gum trouble, and eventually tooth loss.

Step 4

Dialog（和訳）

アンディー先生：どれくらいの頻度で歯を磨きますか？
患者：1日に1回は…でも時々歯を磨かないまま寝てしまいます。
アンディー先生：1回の歯磨きにどれくらい時間をかけていますか？
患者：分かりません。いつもネットをしながらなので。
アンディー先生：うーん。口腔ケアに関してもっと真剣になるべきですよ。
患者：なぜですか？

患者：口の中がとても痛くて、話しづらいわ。
アンディー先生：どこが問題か見てみましょう。口を大きく開けてください。
患者：それで、どうなっているの？
アンディー先生：口内炎ができているみたいですね。
患者：原因は？

モデルエッセイ

　Inflammation or sores of the cheeks, tongue, lips, or gums is called stomatitis. It is a painful condition which gets in the way of eating and talking. Stomatitis has three causes: lack of sleep, trauma, and unbalanced nutrition.

　First, lack of sleep may become the cause of stomatitis. It is important to get enough sleeping hours. Second, stomatitis can be caused by external trauma such as cheek biting or a punch to the face. Third, lack of vitamin B (unbalanced nutrition) can cause stomatitis. It is important to take red meat, salmon, avocado, and bananas.

　In conclusion, stomatitis can be caused by lack of sleep, external trauma, and poor eating habits. It is necessary to have a regular daily life. Of course, regular checkups at the dentist are also important.

（モデルエッセイ和訳）
　頬、舌、唇や歯茎の炎症は口内炎と呼ばれています。食事や会話の邪魔をする痛みを伴う症状です。口内炎の3つの原因は、睡眠不足、外傷そしてバランスの悪い栄養（栄養摂取障害）です。まず、睡眠不足は口内炎の原因になることがあります。十分な睡眠時間を確保することは大切です。次に、口内炎は咬頬（咬舌・咬唇）や顔面へのパンチなどの外傷によって引き起こされることがあります。次に、ビタミンB群不足が口内炎の原因となることがあります。肉の赤身、鮭、アボカドやバナナを摂取することが大切です。従って、口内炎は睡眠不足、外傷そしてよくない食習慣によって起きます。規則正しい生活をする必要があります。もちろん、歯科医院での定期健診も大切です。

患者：考えてみると、ジャンクフードを食べすぎていたわ。
アンディー先生：睡眠の方は？
患者：あまり眠れていないの。
アンディー先生：口内炎用のパッチを処方しておきますね。しっかりと睡眠をとって、栄養のあるものを食べるようにしてください。
患者：わかりました。

Lesson 7. 悪い歯磨きの結果
Step 1

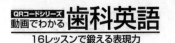

患者：少なくとも歯周病ではなかったみたいですね。

アンディー先生：ええ。でも日々のケアにもう少し注意を払う必要がありますよ。

患者：手始めに、ちゃんとした歯磨きの仕方を教えていただけませんか。

アンディー先生：もちろん。衛生士を呼んできます。

患者：（うれしそう）

Lesson 6. 口内炎の原因

Step 1

1. inflammation 炎症　2. sore / stomatitis 口内炎　3. get in the way 邪魔をする

4. lack of sleep 睡眠不足　5. trauma 外傷

6. unbalanced nutrition バランスの悪い栄養摂取　7. sleeping hours 睡眠時間

8. external 外因性　9. cheek biting 咬頬　10. lack of vitamin ビタミン不足

11. regular daily life 規則正しい生活　12. regular checkups 定期検診

Step 2

Cause 1: lack of sleep

Cause 2: external trauma

　　　　　For example: cheek biting, a punch to the face

Cause 3: unbalanced nutrition, lack of vitamin B

　　　　　For example: red meat, salmon, avocado, bananas

Step 3

Thesis statement:

　Stomatitis has three causes: lack of sleep, trauma, and unbalanced nutrition.

Body:

　1. Lack of sleep may become the cause of stomatitis.

　2. Stomatitis can be caused by external trauma.

　3. Unbalanced nutrition can cause stomatitis.

Conclusion:

　Stomatitis can be caused by lack of sleep, external trauma, and poor eating habits.

Step 4

Dialog（和訳）

アンディー先生：どうされました？

Thesis statement:

There are three causes for bad breath.

Body:

1. Food can be the cause of bad breath.
2. Poor oral care can be a cause of bad breath.
3. Bad breath might be a sign of oral diseases.

Conclusion:

Bad breath is caused by food, lack of care, and oral diseases.

Step 4

Dialog（和訳）

アンディー先生：何これ！

患者：え、どうしましたか？

アンディー先生：お昼に何を食べましたか？

患者：チーズバーガーとオニオンリングですが。それが何か？

アンディー先生：息がかなり玉葱臭いです。

患者：オニオンリングのせいでしょうか？

アンディー先生：あるいはそれ以外のものかも。見ましょう。

モデルエッセイ

　It is quite displeasing when someone nearby has bad breath. There are three causes of bad breath. First, food can be the cause of bad breath. Strong smelling food like cheese, onion, and garlic can make breath smell foul. Next, poor oral care can be a cause of bad breath. Insufficient tooth brushing and lack of flossing can influence the breath. Finally, bad breath might be a sign of oral diseases. Conditions such as cavities and periodontitis make breath smell bad. In conclusion, bad breath is caused by food, lack of care, and oral diseases. It is necessary to have proper knowledge about the causes. Regular checkups at the dental clinic can prevent bad breath.

（モデルエッセイ和訳）

　傍にいる人の口臭が臭いと不快な気分になります。(歯科に関連する)口臭には3つの原因があります。まず、食べ物が口臭を引き起こすことがあります。チーズ、玉ねぎやニンニクなどの強いにおいの食べ物は息を臭くします。次に、よくないお口の手入が口臭を引き起こすことがあります。不十分な歯磨きやフロスの怠りは息に影響を与えます。最後に、歯科疾患を発症している可能性があります。虫歯や歯周炎などの病状は口臭を引き起こします。従って、口臭は食物、ケアの怠りそして歯科疾患によって引き起こされます。原因について正しい知識を持つことが必要です。歯科医院での定期健診は口臭を予防することができます。

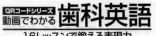

Fourth, a dead tooth can cause discoloration. This condition called necrosis occurs when the pulp is dead. In conclusion, tooth stains have four causes. They are smoking, food, drinks, and dead teeth. Self-care and professional care at a dental clinic are necessary to prevent tooth stains.

（モデルエッセイ和訳）
　歯に着色がついていると恥をかくことがあります。歯の着色には4つの原因があります。まず、喫煙は着色を引き起こすことがあります。煙草に含まれているタールやニコチンが歯を変色させます。次に、食べ物が着色を引き起こすことがあります。チョコレートやカレーのように色素を含む食物は歯を変色させます。次に、飲み物が着色の原因となることがある。コーヒーやワインのようにタンニンを含む飲み物は歯を変色させる。次に、死んだ歯が変色を引き起こすことがある。壊死と呼ばれるこの状態は歯髄が死んだ時に起きる。従って、歯の着色には4つの原因があります。それらは、喫煙、食物、飲料、そして死活歯です。歯の着色を予防するためにはセルフケアと歯科医院でのケアが必要です。

（治療後）
患者：（鏡を見て）すごい！全く違う。
アンディー先生：さあ、これで面接に向けて準備万端ですね。
患者：何か面接の秘訣はありますか？
アンディー先生：笑顔を忘れずに。あなたの綺麗な歯を面接官たちに見せつけてやることかな。

Lesson 5. 口臭の原因

Step 1
1. displeasing 不快　2. bad breath 口臭　3. strong smelling 臭いのきつい
4. smell foul 嫌な臭いがする　5. poor よくない　6. oral care 口腔ケア
7. insufficient 不十分な　8. lack of〜不足　9. flossing フロス　10. influence 影響する
11. oral disease 口腔疾患　12. periodontitis 歯周炎　13. proper 正しい
14. knowledge 知識　15. regular checkups 定期検診　16. prevent 予防

Step 2
Cause 1: food (eating habits)
　　　　　for example: cheese, onion, garlic
Cause 2: poor oral care
　　　　　for example: insufficient tooth brushing, lack of flossing
Cause 3: oral disease
　　　　　for example: cavities, gum trouble

Step 3

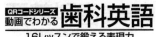

Plaque is formed by bacteria which feed on sugar.

Lesson 4. 歯の着色の原因

Step 1

1. stains 着色 2. embarrassing 恥ずかしい 3. smoking 喫煙 4. tar タール
5. nicotine ニコチン 6. tobacco タバコ 7. discolor 変色させる 8. pigment 色素
9. tannin タンニン 10. dead tooth 死歯 11. discoloration 変色 12. necrosis 壊死
13. pulp 歯髄 14. self care セルフケア 15. professional care 歯科医師などによるケア

Step 2

1. smoking
2. food 例えば chocolate, curry
3. drinks 例えば coffee, wine
4. dead tooth

Step 3

Thesis statement:
　There are four causes to tooth stains.

Body（省略）

Conclusion:
　Tooth stains have four causes. They are smoking, food, drinks, and dead teeth.

Step 4

Dialog（和訳）

患者：アンディー先生、最終の採用面接までたどり着きました。

アンディー先生：それは朗報ですね！でも、残念なお知らせもあります。

患者：何でしょうか。

アンディー先生：歯にかなりのステインが付いています。

患者：(鏡を見て) うわ！

モデルエッセイ

　Having stains on your teeth can be embarrassing. There are four causes of tooth stains. First, smoking can cause stains. The tar and nicotine contained in tobacco discolors the teeth. Second, food can cause stains. Food that contain pigments such as chocolate and curry can discolor teeth. Third, drinks can be a cause of stains. Drinks that contain tannin such as coffee and wine discolor the teeth.

アンディー先生：凹凸や角はありますか。
患者：いいえ。とても滑らかだわ。
アンディー先生：そうですか。では終了です。
患者：いつから食べてもいいかしら？
アンディー先生：1時間ほど待ってください。

II. Cause & Effect—原因と結果を説明してみよう！（Lesson 4～7）

Step 1
結果を表す単語やフレーズ：

1. ～という結果になる（r、2語で）
   result in
2. 結果として（a、3語で）
   as a result
3. したがって（t）
   therefore
4. したがって（t）
   thus
5. したがって（c）
   consequently
6. したがって（h）
   hence
7. したがって（s）
   so
8. したがって（t）
   thereby

原因を表す単語やフレーズ：

1. ～というのは（f）
   for
2. なぜなら（b）
   because
3. なぜなら（s）
   since
4. なぜなら（a）
   as
5. ～が原因で（d, 2語で）
   due to
6. ～が原因で（o, 3語で）
   on account of
7. ～によって（b）
   by

Step 2
1. 激しい歯磨きは歯茎のダメージにつながりうる。
   Brushing too hard can result in damage to the gums.
2. 私は食べ過ぎた。その結果、私のジーンズはきつい。
   I ate too much. As a result, my jeans are tight.
3. 口臭はニンニクの入った食べ物が多すぎることが原因だ。
   Bad breath is due to eating too much food with garlic.
4. 歯垢は砂糖をエサとする細菌によって形成される。

Step 2
1. Apply local anesthetic to the gums.
2. Drill away the decayed parts.
3. Fill with composite resin.
4. Shine light on the resin to harden.
5. Polish the surface.

Step 3

Thesis statement:

There are five steps in treating cavities.

Body（省略）

Conclusion:

This is how to treat cavities.

Step 4

Dialog（和訳）

（患者の口をのぞき込み）

アンディー先生：虫歯があるみたいですね。

患者：おかしいわね。全く痛みを感じないけど。

アンディー先生：まだ初期段階の虫歯です。

患者：どうしたらいいかしら？

アンディー先生：痛くなり始める前に治療をおすすめします。

患者：どのように治療するのかしら？

モデルエッセイ：

There are five steps in treating cavities. First, apply local anesthetic to the gums. Check if the anesthetic has taken effect. Second, drill away the decayed parts. Third, fill with composite resin. Fourth, shine light on the resin to harden. Finally, polish the surface. So, this is how to treat cavities.

（モデルエッセイ和訳）

虫歯の治療には5つの手順があります。まず、歯茎に局所麻酔を注射します。麻酔が利いているか確認します。次に虫歯の部分を削り取ります。次にレジンという詰めものを入れます。次にレジンに光を照射して固めます。最後に表面を磨きます。このようにして虫歯の治療を行います。

アンディー先生：歯に沿って舌を動かしてみてください。

患者：はい。

Dialog（和訳）

（染め出し中）

アンディー先生：この鏡を持ってください。

患者：（鏡を見て）うわ！

アンディー先生：青い箇所が磨き損ねた歯垢を示しています。

患者：十分に歯を磨いたと思いました。

アンディー先生：では、歯の磨き方を教えます。お口をゆすいでください。

モデルエッセイ

　I will explain how to brush your teeth. There are six steps. First, choose a toothbrush with soft bristles. Second, hold the toothbrush with a pen grip. Third, apply the toothbrush to the tooth surface at a 90-degree angle and brush with short strokes. Fourth, apply the toothbrush to the gums at a 45-degree angle and brush with short strokes. Brush the outer, inner, and chewing surfaces of the teeth. Finally, tilt the brush vertically for the inside of the front teeth. So, this is how to brush your teeth.

（モデルエッセイ和訳）

　歯の磨き方を説明します。6つの手順があります。まず、柔らかい毛先の歯ブラシを選んでください。次に、ペンを持つように歯ブラシを持ってください。次に、歯面に対して90度の角度で歯ブラシを当て小さい動きで磨いてください。次に、歯茎に対して45度の角度で歯ブラシを当て小さい動きで磨いてください。歯の外側、内側そして噛む面を磨いてください。最後に前歯の内側を磨くために歯ブラシを垂直に立てください。このようにして歯を磨きます。

アンディー先生：（彼に鏡を見せて）いかがですか？

患者：おお！まったく違います。

アンディー先生：飲み込みが早いですね。

患者：これからはテレビを見ずに歯磨きに集中します。

アンディー先生：その調子です！

Lesson 3. 虫歯の治療の仕方

Step 1

1. cavity 虫歯　2. apply 注射する　3. local anesthetic 局所麻酔　4. check 確認する
5. anesthetic 麻酔薬　6. take effect 効く（効果を現す）　7. drill away 削り取る
8. decay う蝕　9. fill 充填する　10. composite resin (cement) コンポジットレジン
11. shine（光を）当てる　12. harden 固める　13. polish 磨く

に、右に曲がって道沿いに歩いてください。次に、美容院の角で左に曲がってください。道に沿ってまっすぐ進んでください。次にコンビニの前を通り過ぎてください。その後、26号線で左に曲がってください。1分ほど歩いてください。歯科医院は左側にあります。このようにして歯科医院へ来ていただきます。道に迷いましたら遠慮なくお電話ください。

（クリニックの入り口で）
アンディー先生：たどり着きましたね。
患者：そうですね。あなたの説明は適格でした。
アンディー先生：では、始めましょうか？
患者：ええ。
アンディー先生：スリッパに履き替えてください。さあ、こちらへ。

Lesson 2. 歯磨きの仕方

Step 1

1. brush 磨く 2. bristles 毛先 3. apply 当てる 4. tooth surface 歯面
5. 90 degree angle ９０度の角度 6. short strokes 小さい動き
7. 45 degree angle ４５度の角度 8. outer surface 外側の面 9. inner surface 内側の面
10. chewing surface 噛む面 11. tilt 傾ける 12. vertically 垂直に

Step 2

1. Choose a toothbrush with soft bristles.
2. Hold the toothbrush with a pen grip.
3. Apply the toothbrush to the tooth surface at a 90 degree angle and brush with short strokes.
4. Apply the toothbrush to the gums at a 45 degree angle and brush with short strokes.
5. Brush the outer, inner, and chewing surfaces of the teeth.
6. Tilt the brush vertically for the inside of the front teeth.

Step 3

Thesis statement:
　I will explain how to brush your teeth. There are six steps.
Body（省略）
Conclusion:
　This is how to brush your teeth.

Step 4

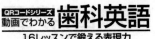

Step 2

1. Go out <u>from the west exit of the station.</u>
2. Turn <u>right and walk along the street.</u>
3. Turn <u>left at the beauty parlor.</u>
4. Go <u>straight along the street.</u>
5. Go <u>past the convenience store.</u>
6. Turn <u>left at Route 26.</u>
7. Walk <u>straight for about 1 minute.</u>
8. The clinic is <u>on the left side.</u>

Step 3

Thesis statement:
　I will explain how to go to the dental clinic from the station. It takes about 5 minutes.

Body（省略）

Conclusion:
　This is how to go to the dental clinic. Don't hesitate to phone us if you get lost.

Step 4

Dialog（和訳）

患者：もしもし？アンディー歯科クリニックですか？
アンディー先生：はい。私がアンディーです。
患者：あなたのクリニックを探していますが、迷ったようです。
アンディー先生：今はどこにいますか？
患者：駅にいます。
アンディー先生：分かりました。今から道順をお伝えします。

モデルエッセイ：

　I will explain how to go to the dental clinic from the station. It takes about 5 minutes. First, go out from the west exit of the station. Second, turn right and walk along the street. Third, turn left at the beauty parlor. Fourth, go straight along the street. Fifth, go past the convenience store. Next, turn left at Route 26. Then, walk straight for about 1 minute. Finally, the clinic is on the left side. So, this is how to go to the dental clinic. Don't hesitate to phone us if you get lost.

（モデルエッセイ和訳）

　駅から歯科医院までの道順を説明します。5分ほどかかります。まず、駅の西口から出てください。次

Answers

Lesson 0. アウトラインとは？

Step 1

1. first　（　最初に　）
2. second　（　二番目に　）
3. third　（　三番目に　）
4. finally　（　最後に　）
5. for example　（　例えば　）
6. for instance　（　例えば　）
7. in conclusion　（　結論として　）
8. therefore　（　したがって　）
9. favorite　（　一番好きな　）
10. reason　（　理由　）
11. because　（　なぜなら　）
12. there is [are] ~　（　～がある　）

I. Process —過程を説明してみよう！（Lesson 1～3）

Step 1

1. まず　first
2. 次に　next
3. 2番目に　second
4. 3番目に　third
5. それから (t)　then
6. そして (a)　and
7. 最後に (f)　finally
8. 最後に (l)　last
9. 結論として（2語で）in conclusion

Step 2

1. まず、バス停まで歩きます。
   First, walk to the bus stop.
2. 次にバスに乗って、そして京都駅で降ります。
   Next, take a (the) bus and get off at Kyoto Station.
3. 3番目に、京都駅で電車に乗ります。
   Third, get on a (the) train at Kyoto Station.
4. それから、大阪駅で地下鉄に乗り換えます。
   Then, change to the subway at Osaka Station.
5. 最後に、難波駅で降りてください。
   Finally, get off at Namba Station.

Lesson 1. 駅から歯科医院までの道順

Step 1

Go <u>straight</u>.　　　　　　　　　Go <u>straight for 50 meters</u>.
Turn <u>right</u>.　　　　　　　　　　Turn <u>right at the first intersection</u>.
Go <u>past</u>.　　　　　　　　　　　Go <u>past the supermarket</u>.
The clinic <u>is on the left</u>.　　　　You will find <u>the clinic in front of you</u>.

QRコードシリーズ 動画でわかる 歯科英語

16レッスンで鍛える表現力

〈解答集〉

浪速社

Lesson 5
The causes of bad breath

> STEP 4　英語で言ってみよう！

1．モデルエッセイでシャドーイングをしなさい。
2．現場での使われ方を **Dialog** で確認しよう。

Dialog
Andy: Oh my god!
Patient: Oh my god, what?
Andy: What did you have for lunch?
Patient: A cheese burger and some onion rings. Why?
Andy: Your breath smells strongly of onions.
Patient: Could it be the onion rings?
Andy: Or something else. Let's take a look.

モデルエッセイ： **The causes of bad breath**

(following the checkup)
Patient: At least it wasn't gum disease.
Andy: Yes, but you have to be more careful with your daily care.
Patient: To start, could you teach me how to brush properly?
Andy: Sure. I'll get my hygienist.
Patient:　（うれしそう）

Try this in English 応用編　アウトラインを作成して英語でプレゼンしよう。

タイトル　I have good / poor oral health

1．＿＿＿＿＿＿＿＿＿＿＿＿＿＿＿＿＿＿＿＿＿

2．＿＿＿＿＿＿＿＿＿＿＿＿＿＿＿＿＿＿＿＿＿

3．＿＿＿＿＿＿＿＿＿＿＿＿＿＿＿＿＿＿＿＿＿　　注：必ず具体例(for example)をつける。

Lesson 6. 口内炎の原因

The causes of stomatitis

Message from Dr. Andy

Mouth sores are a cause of discomfort when eating and talking. My patients seem quite happy when this problem is resolved speedily. People are not aware that improper tooth brushing can also be a cause.

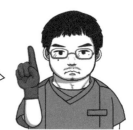

STEP 1　必要な単語の確認

次の語を和訳してみよう。

1. inflammation
2. sore / stomatitis
3. get in the way

4. lack of sleep
5. trauma
6. unbalanced nutrition

7. sleeping hours
8. external
9. cheek biting

10. lack of vitamin
11. regular daily life
12. regular checkups

Lesson 6
The causes of stomatitis

STEP 2　英語で書いてみよう！

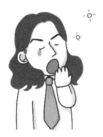

Cause 1　（睡眠不足）_____

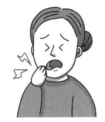 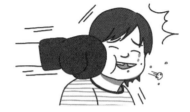

Cause 2　（外傷）_____

　　For example, _____

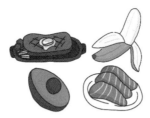

Cause 3　（バランスの悪い食事）_____

　　　　（ビタミンB不足）_____

　　For example, <u>take</u>_____

Lesson 6
The causes of stomatitis

> STEP 3　アウトラインを作成する

OUTLINE

Thesis statement（主題）「口内炎には睡眠不足、外傷、バランスの悪い食事の3つの原因がある。」

Body（本文）（3つの原因を簡潔に書きだそう）

1.

2.

3.

Conclusion（結論）「口内炎は睡眠不足、外傷、バランスの悪い食事によって引き起こされる。」

アウトラインをもとにエッセイを書いたら、QRコードを読み取って一休み

Lesson 6
The causes of stomatitis

STEP 4 英語で言ってみよう！

1．モデルエッセイでシャドーイングをしなさい。
2．現場での使われ方を **Dialog** で確認しよう。

Dialog

Andy: What seems to be the problem?

Patient: The inside of my mouth hurts so much I even have trouble talking.

Andy: Let's see what is wrong. Open wide.

Patient: So what's happening?

Andy: You seem to have canker sores.

Patient: What is the cause?

モデルエッセイ： **The causes of stomatitis**

Patient: Come to think of it, I've been eating too much junk food.

Andy: What about sleep?

Patient: Not much.

Andy: I will prescribe some patches for your condition. Be sure to get some sleep and some nutrition.

Patient: Okay.

Try this in English 応用編　アウトラインを作成して英語でプレゼンしよう。

タイトル　What kind of dentist would you like to be?

1．_____

2．_____

3．_____

注：重要度の順で並べるように。

Lesson 7
The effects of poor tooth brushing

Lesson 7. 悪い歯磨きの結果

The effects of poor tooth brushing

Message from Dr. Andy

Oral health is being promoted through the 80-20 campaign which aims for 20 teeth at the age of 80. However, even if that many teeth remain, years of improper brushing can deteriorate their condition.

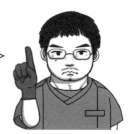

STEP 1　必要な単語の確認

次の語を日本語に直しなさい。

1. poor tooth brushing
2. negative
3. oral health

4. tooth stains
5. tooth decay
6. plaque

7. build up
8. attack
9. tooth enamel

10. bring about
11. gum trouble
12. bacteria

13. as a result of
14. tooth loss
15. occur

16. eventually
17. assessment

Lesson 7
The effects of poor tooth brushing

STEP 2　英語で書いてみよう！

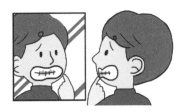

Effect 1　（着色）：

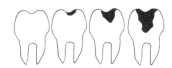

Effect 2　（う蝕）：

（プラークが蓄積してエナメル質を侵食する）：

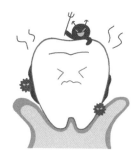

Effect 3　（歯肉のトラブル）：

（細菌が歯肉の下に蓄積する）：

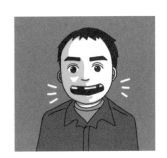

Effect 4　（歯の喪失）：

（う蝕やガムトラブルにより歯の喪失が起きる）：

Lesson 7
The effects of poor tooth brushing

STEP 3　アウトラインを作成する

OUTLINE

Thesis statement（主題）「悪い歯磨きは４つの良くない結果を導く。」

Body（本文）（４つの結果を簡潔に書きだそう）

1.

2.

3.

4.

Conclusion（結論）「悪い歯磨きは、着色、う蝕、歯肉のトラブル、そして歯の喪失につながる。」

アウトラインをもとにエッセイを書いたら、QRコードを読み取って一休み

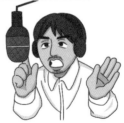

Lesson 7
The effects of poor tooth brushing

STEP 4 英語で言ってみよう！

1. モデルエッセイでシャドーイングをしなさい。
2. 現場での使われ方を **Dialog** で確認しよう。

> Dialog
> (oral care interview)
> Andy: How often do you brush your teeth?
> Patient: Once a day...sometimes I just fall asleep without brushing.
> Andy: How much time do you spend on each brushing?
> Patient: I don't know. I'm always surfing the Net.
> Andy: Hmmm. You should be more serious about your oral care.
> Patient: Why is that?
>
> モデルエッセイ： The effects of poor tooth brushing
>
> Patient: Oh boy! Sounds like a horror story.
> Andy: My hygienist will teach you how to brush properly.
> Patient: (Looking toward a cute young assistant) Right away!
> Hygienist: (a guy appears from a different angle)
>   Hi. I am your hygienist!

Try this in English 応用編　アウトラインを作成して英語でプレゼンしよう。
タイトル　The effects of healthy white teeth

1. _____
2. _____
3. _____

II Cause and Effect

III. Definition—定義づけて説明してみよう！
（Lesson 8～9）

Definition は物事を定義しながら説明をする方法である。ケンブリッジのオンライン辞書で toothpaste を調べると "a thick, creamy substance that you put on a toothbrush to clean your teeth" と定義づけられている。順番としては、まず単語が属しているカテゴリー（分野）を説明する。Toothpaste の場合は、「濃いクリーム状の物質」となる。関係代名詞の that を挟んで特徴である「歯をきれいにするために歯ブラシにつける」が続く。

Definition は、日本のことを知らない外国人に日本の伝統的な物を説明する時に役立つ。例えば "What is natto?" と尋ねられるとどう返事をするだろう。多くの場合、慌てて「ネバネバした」とか「においが強い」などの特徴を英訳しょうとする。聞く側には、極めて分かりにくい説明になる。まずは、カテゴリである "traditional Japanese food"（伝統的な日本の食べ物）であることを伝える。関係代名詞の "which" を挟んで特徴である "is fermented soy beans（発酵した大豆）mixed with soy sauce, green onions, and mustard（醤油、ネギ、からしと混ぜる）. It is eaten with steamed rice（ご飯と一緒に食べる）...." と続く。特徴の長さや内容は自由である。納豆嫌いの人は "terrible smell"（ひどいにおい）や "very sticky"（とてもネチネチしている）を使って独断と偏見で定義付けする楽しさもある。

歯科医院では外国人患者に器具などの説明をする時に定義付けを使うことができる。
ラバーダム is a piece of rubber that is used to keep the teeth dry during dental treatment.
印象材 is a material that helps take accurate impressions of the teeth.

本章ではパラグラフ単位の定義付けを取り上げる。

> STEP 1　英語で書いてみよう！

以下の各英文を読んで、それぞれが何を定義しているか英語で書きなさい。

1．The largest mammal that lives in the sea

2．A room in which meals are cooked or prepared

3．A natural flow of water that continues in a long line across land to the ocean

4．A small creature with eight thin legs which spins webs to catch insects for food

5．A piece of body tissue that you tighten and relax to move a particular part of the body

> STEP 2　英語で定義してみよう！

以下の各語を英語で定義しなさい。

1．ゾウ

2．10月

3．地球

4．バナナ

5．歯科医師

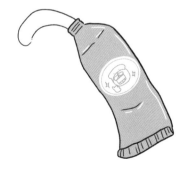

Lesson 8. 美しい笑顔とは

Definition of a beautiful smile

Message from Dr. Andy

A set of healthy teeth is the minimum requirement for a beautiful smile. If you are not confident in your oral health, visit a dentist right away. Our job is to restore that beautiful smile.

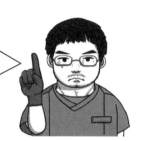

STEP 1　必要な単語の確認

次の語を日本語に直しなさい。

1. confidence
2. factor
3. teeth alignment

4. facial expression
5. orthodontic treatment
6. crooked teeth

7. irregular
8. whitening treatment
9. convey

10. rich

Lesson 8
Definition of a beautiful smile

STEP 2 英語で書いてみよう！

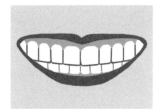

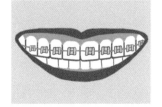

1. （歯並び）

具体的に：（矯正によって歯並びや咬合を治すことができる）

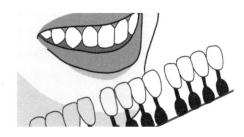

2. （歯の色）

具体的に：（ホワイトニングは色のついた歯を白くしてくれる）

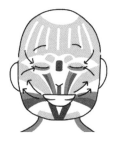

3. （顔の表情）

具体的に：（豊かな表情で気持ちを表す）

Lesson 8
Definition of a beautiful smile

STEP 3　アウトラインを作成する

OUTLINE

Thesis statement（主題）　　「美しい笑顔には3つの要素がある。」

Body（本文）（3つの要素を英語で書きなさい。）

1.

2.

3.

Conclusion（結論）「美しい笑顔のための3つの要素は良い歯並びと良い歯の色と豊かな表情である。」

アウトラインをもとにエッセイを書いたら、QRコードを読み取って一休み

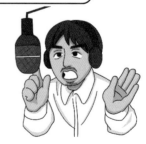

Lesson 8
Definition of a beautiful smile

STEP 4 英語で言ってみよう！

1. モデルエッセイでシャドーイングをしなさい。
2. 現場での使われ方をDialogで確認しよう。

Dialog
Mutti: That's a cool tie you have on there.
Patient: Thanks. I just bought a whole set of new suits.
Mutti: Changing your image?
Patient: Yes, with my new job....I wonder if there is anything else I can do.
Mutti: How about your smile?
Patient: My smile?

モデルエッセイ： **Definition of a beautiful smile**

Patient: A beautiful smile will surely help my new work.
Mutti: Would you like to try whitening?
Patient: Right away.
Mutti: You can start by taking this tie off.

Try this in English 応用編　アウトラインを作成して英語でプレゼンしよう。
タイトル　Definition of a delicious bowl of ramen　美味しいラーメンとは
(他、好きな食べ物で)

1. _____

2. _____

3. _____　　注：3つの要素（factors）を説明する。

Lesson 9
Definition of a good dentist

Lesson 9. 良い歯科医とは

Definition of a good dentist

Message from Dr. Andy

I always make sure to place my patient's interests first. Also, it is important to respect their dignity. Good communication skills and of course, treatment skills are essential. Oh, and don't forget, English!

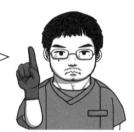

STEP 1　必要な単語の確認

次の語を和訳してみよう。

1. good
2. qualities
3. communication skills

4. respect
5. firm
6. skills

7. establish
8. rapport
9. in turn

10. dentistry
11. question / inquiry
12. regain

Lesson 9
Definition of a good dentist

STEP 2　英語で書いてみよう！

1.　（コミュニケーション能力）

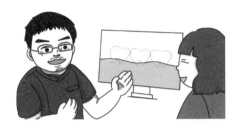

2.　（患者に対する尊敬の気持ち）

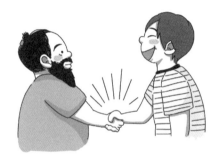

3.　（知識）

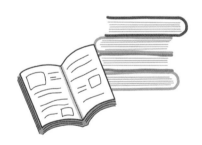

4.　（技術）

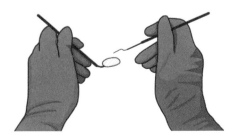

Lesson 9
Definition of a good dentist

STEP 3　アウトラインを作成する

OUTLINE

Thesis statement（主題）「よい歯科医師には４つの特質がある」

Body（本文）（４つの特質を英語で書きなさい。）

1.

2.

3.

4.

Conclusion（結論）　「良い歯科医師はコミュニケーション能力があり、患者を尊敬し、知識があり、技術を持っている。」

アウトラインをもとにエッセイを書いたら、QRコードを読み取って一休み

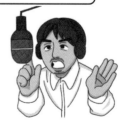

Lesson 9
Definition of a good dentist

STEP 4 英語で言ってみよう！

1．モデルエッセイでシャドーイングをしなさい。
2．現場での使われ方を **Dialog** で確認しよう。

Dialog
　(at a coffee shop)
Sally: Do you always go to the same dentist?
Jerry: Sure. I visit this guy regularly for checkups.
Sally: Does he speak good English?
Jerry: He is quite fluent...not only that, he is....

モデルエッセイ：　Definition of a good dentist

Sally: Sounds like a good dentist.
Jerry: Actually, his clinic is right around the corner.
Sally: Really? Could you show me where it is?
Jerry: Sure, why not. Let's....(Dr. Andy is in the background drinking coffee)
Andy: Hello. Sally? This way please. (the two leave)
Jerry: (notices and picks up the check)

Try this in English 応用編　アウトラインを作成して英語でプレゼンしよう。
タイトル　Definition of a popular guy/gal　　異性にモテる男・女

1．_____

2．_____

3．_____　　注：3つの特質（qualities）を説明する。

IV. Comparison―比較して説明してみよう！
（Lesson 10～13）

Comparisonは２つの物事を比較して相違点もしくは類似点を明らかにする説明の仕方である。歯科医院を訪れた外国人患者には治療の選択肢を分かりやすく説明するのに使うことができる。

鉛筆とシャープペンを比較するとしよう。まずは、"I will explain the differences between pencils and mechanical pencils"（これから鉛筆とシャープペンの違いを説明します）と説明の主題を伝える。次に<u>重さ</u>、<u>価格</u>、書き味など比較の項目をつけて具体的な違いを明らかにする。例えば、"The first difference is <u>weight</u>. Pencils are extremely light while mechanical pencils are slightly heavier. The second difference is <u>cost</u>...."（まず最初に重さが異なる。鉛筆はとても軽い。それに対し、シャープペンは少し重さがある。二つ目の違いは価格である、、、）のように説明していく。

比較の項目が上記の３つに加え、強度、デザイン性、持ち運び、エコ、、、と多い場合は説明が単調になる可能性がある。その場合、「鉛筆は、、、シャーペンは、、、鉛筆は、、、シャーペンは、、、」と交互に説明するのではなく、鉛筆の説明をまとめて一気にする。そのあとシャープペンの説明を続ける。鉛筆及びシャープペンの説明をする時の項目の内容と順番が同じでなければならない。

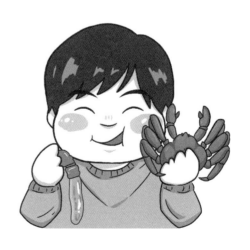

STEP 1　必要な単語の確認

次の語を英語に直しなさい。括弧が与えられている場合は、そのアルファベットから始めること。

相違点：

1．対照的に（i、2語で）　　　　　　2．一方で（o、4語で）

3．しかしながら（h）　　　　　　　4．一方で（w）

5．一方で（w）　　　　　　　　　　6．しかし（b）

7．しかし（y）

類似点：

1．同様に（l）　　　　　　　　　　2．同様に（s）

3．さらに（a）　　　　　　　　　　4．～とおり（j、2語で）

5．～と～ともに（b）

STEP 2　英語で書いてみよう！

1．リンゴは赤い。しかしながら、バナナは黄色い。

2．アメリカ合衆国は大きな国である一方で、日本は小さい。

3．コーヒーは山で栽培される。同様に、お茶も高地で栽培される。

4．ロシアは中国もそうである通り大きな国だ。

Lesson 10. 日本と豪州の歯学部の違い

The difference between dental schools of Japan and Australia

Message from Dr. Andy

If there is a chance to visit a dental school abroad, I strongly recommend that you go. It is a way to broaden your perspectives. Not only that, wouldn't it be cool to have a bunch of dentist friends around the globe?

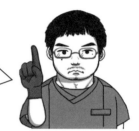

STEP 1　必要な単語の確認

次の語を日本語に直しなさい。

1. dental school

2. differences

3. high school graduate

4. apply for

5. college graduate

6. BA

7. six year course

8. clinics

9. graduate

10. national board examination

11. licensed dentist

12. upon graduation

Lesson 10
The differences between dental schools of Japan and Australia

STEP 2　英語で書いてみよう！

日本の歯学部：

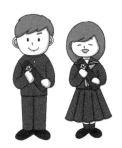

１．受験者： 　　　　　　　　　　２．就学年数：

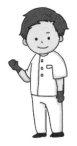

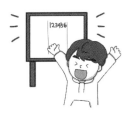

３．臨床実習開始年次： 　　　　　４．資格取得：

オーストラリアの歯学部：

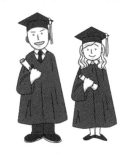

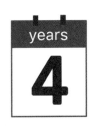

１．受験者： 　　　　　　　　　　２．就学年数：

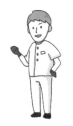

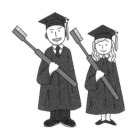

３．臨床実習開始年次： 　　　　　４．資格取得：

Lesson 10
The differences between dental schools of Japan and Australia

STEP 3　アウトラインを作成する

OUTLINE

Thesis statement（主題）「日本とオーストラリアの歯学部の間には4つの違いがある。」

Body（本文）　（表の空欄を埋めよう）

何を比較するか　↓	Japan	Australia
1. 受験者		
2. 就学年数		
3. 臨床実習開始年次		
4. 資格取得		

Conclusion（結論）「日本とオーストラリアの歯学部の間には主に4つの違いがある。」

アウトラインをもとにエッセイを書いたら、QR コードを読み取って一休み

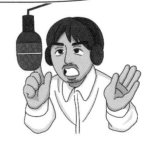

Lesson 10
The differences between dental schools of Japan and Australia

STEP 4　英語で言ってみよう！

1．モデルエッセイでシャドーイングをしなさい。
2．現場での使われ方をDialogで確認しよう。

Dialog

Andy: Rinse out your mouth please. This is all for today.
　　　I will see you again next week.
Patient: Thanks. By the way, when did you start practicing here?
Andy: After I passed the board exam...about 10 years ago.
Patient: You have to take a test after you graduate?
Andy: In order to get a license, yes.
Patient: My friend in Sydney graduated and started seeing patients right away.
Andy: The system is different between Japan and Australia.

モデルエッセイ：　The difference between dental schools of Japan and Australia

Patient: I see. In either country, becoming a dentist requires hard work.
Andy: Yes, but it is a satisfying job especially when you see your patient smiling.
Patient: Like this? (smiles)
Andy: Yes...and you still haven't rinsed out your mouth.

Try this in English 応用編　アウトラインを作成して英語でプレゼンしよう。

タイトル　食べ物の比較（同じジャンルであること「きのこの@」と「たけのこの@」など。

比較の項目↓	きのこの@	たけのこの@
形		
食感		
味		

Lesson 11
The differences between metal crowns and ceramic crowns

Lesson 11. メタルクラウンとセラミッククラウンの違い

The difference between metal crowns and ceramic crowns

Message from Dr. Andy

Once a crown is placed, it is not so easy to remove. That is why the decision process is important. It is necessary to take into consideration, the appearance, the occlusion, and in some cases, the budget.

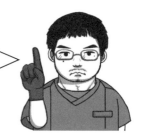

STEP 1　必要な単語の確認

次の語を和訳してみよう。

1. insured

2. not insured

3. metallic

4. appearance

5. natural

6. durable

7. crack

8. allergy

Lesson 11

The differences between metal crowns and ceramic crowns

STEP 2　英語で書いてみよう！

メタルクラウン：

1．保険適用：

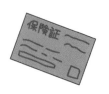

2．見た目：

3．強度：

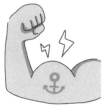

4．アレルギー反応

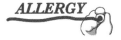

セラミッククラウン：

1．保険適用：

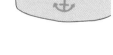

2．見た目：

3．強度

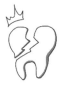

4．アレルギー反応

Lesson 11
The differences between metal crowns and ceramic crowns

STEP 3　アウトラインを作成する

OUTLINE

Thesis statement（主題）「メタルクラウンとセラミッククラウンには４つの違いがある。」

Body（本文）　（表の空欄を埋めよう）

対比の項目↓	metal crown	ceramic crown
1. 保険適用		
2. 見た目		
3. 強度		
4. アレルギー反応		

Conclusion（結論）「メタルクラウンとセラミッククラウンには４つの違いがある。」

アウトラインをもとにエッセイを書いたら、QRコードを読み取って一休み

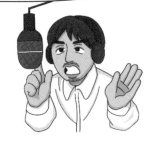

Lesson 11

The differences between metal crowns and ceramic crowns

STEP 4　英語で言ってみよう！

1．モデルエッセイでシャドーイングをしなさい。
2．現場での使われ方を **Dialog** で確認しよう。

Dialog

Andy: I have finished preparing your tooth to attach the crown.

Patient: What is the next procedure?

Andy: We need to choose the type of crown.

Patient: What are the choices?

Andy: You can choose either a metal crown or a ceramic crown.

Patient: What are the differences?

モデルエッセイ： The difference between metal crowns and ceramic crowns

Patient: I guess I will choose metal.

Andy: Good choice. Since it is in the back, the stronger one would be better.

Patient: I hope it won't be visible.

Andy: Just be sure to cover your mouth when yawning.

Try this in English 応用編　アウトラインを作成して英語でプレゼンしよう。

タイトル 紙辞書と電子辞書　（今度は比較の項目を自分で考えよう）

比較の項目↓	紙辞書	電子辞書

IV *Comparison*

Lesson 12
The differences between implants and bridges

Lesson 12. インプラントとブリッジの違い

The difference between implants and bridges

Message from Dr. Andy

Many of my patients wish for immediate results. However, when choosing the type of prosthesis, I make sure to explain what to expect 10 to 20 years later. The decision needs to be based on a balance of the two.

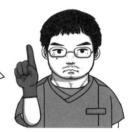

STEP 1　必要な単語の確認

次の語を和訳してみよう。

1. implants
2. bridge
3. strain

4. nearby
5. drilling
6. maintenance

7. require
8. self-care
9. professional care

10. long time
11. short time

Lesson 12
The differences between implants and bridges

STEP 2　英語で書いてみよう！

インプラント：

1．隣接歯への影響

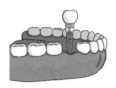

なし：

2．メンテナンス

セルフケア：　　　プロケア：

3．時間

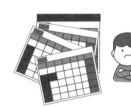

かかる：

4．費用

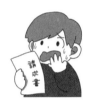

高価：

ブリッジ：

1．隣接歯への影響

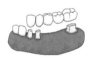

削る：

2．メンテナンス

セルフケア：

3．時間

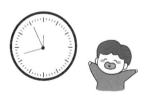

短時間：

4．費用

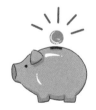

安価：

Lesson 12
The differences between implants and bridges

STEP 3　アウトラインを作成する

OUTLINE

Thesis statement（主題）「インプラントとブリッジには4つの違いがある。」

Body（本文）　（表の空欄を埋めよう）

対比の項目↓	implants	bridges
1.		
2.		
3.		
4.		

Conclusion（結論）「インプラントとブリッジには4つの違いがある。」

アウトラインをもとにエッセイを書いたら、QRコードを読み取って一休み

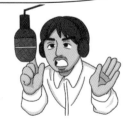

Lesson 12
The differences between implants and bridges

STEP 4　英語で言ってみよう！

1．モデルエッセイでシャドーイングをしなさい。
2．現場での使われ方を **Dialog** で確認しよう。

Dialog

Mutti: It sure was a terrible accident.

Patient: Yes. It is hard to believe that I am still alive.

Mutti: Now we have to do something about the gap between your teeth.

Patient: What kind of treatment is possible?

Mutti: You can have a bridge or an implant.

Patient: What is the difference?

モデルエッセイ： The difference between implants and bridges

Patient: Now this surely is a difficult choice.

Mutti: If you can afford it, I think an implant would be better.

Patient: Yeah, I do not want my other teeth drilled.

Mutti: Okay. If you would come to my office in the back, I will give you more details.

Try this in English 応用編　アウトラインを作成して英語でプレゼンしよう。

タイトル　自由（注意：同じジャンルであることが大事）

比較の項目↓		
1.		
2.		
3.		

Lesson 13
The differences between whitening and veneers

Lesson 13. ホワイトニングとベニアの違い

The difference between whitening and veneers

Message from Dr. Andy

A veneer is a thin layer of porcelain which is placed over the front surface of a tooth. There are conditions that can only be fixed by the use of veneers. Tooth staining caused by Tetracycline is one of them.

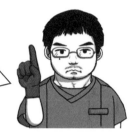

STEP 1　必要な単語の確認

次の語を和訳してみよう。

1. whitening
2. veneer
3. application

4. chemicals
5. porcelain
6. attach

7. invasive
8. drilling
9. cost

10. per treatment
11. in contrast
12. effect

Lesson 13
The differences between whitening and veneers

STEP 2　英語で書いてみよう！

ホワイトニング:

1．方法：

薬品：

2．侵襲性：

削らない：

3．コスト

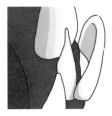

40000円：

4．耐久年数

2〜3年：

ベニア:

1．方法：

接着：

2．侵襲性

削る：

3．コスト

1歯につき100000円

4．耐久年数

5〜10年：

Lesson 13
The differences between whitening and veneers

STEP 3　アウトラインを作成する

OUTLINE

Thesis statement（主題）「ホワイトニングとベニアの治療には４つの違いがある。」

Body（本文）　（表の空欄を埋めよう）

対比の項目↓	whitening	veneer
1.		
2.		
3.		
4.		

Conclusion（結論）「ホワイトニングとベニアの治療には４つの違いがある。」

アウトラインをもとにエッセイを書いたら、QR コードを読み取って一休み

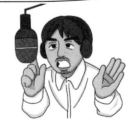

Lesson 13
The differences between whitening and veneers

STEP 4　英語で言ってみよう！

1．モデルエッセイでシャドーイングをしなさい。
2．現場での使われ方を **Dialog** で確認しよう。

Dialog

Patient: I am going to give a presentation to a huge audience.
Andy: Sounds exciting!
Patient: …but, I am a bit worried about my appearance.
Andy: In what way?
Patient: My tooth color….

モデルエッセイ：　The difference between whitening and veneers

Andy: When is the presentation?
Patient: Next month.
Andy: Then, why don't you try whitening?
Patient: OK. I guess the veneers can wait.

Try this in English 応用編

項目別ではなく、ホワイトニングをまとめて説明してからベニアを同じように説明する方法もある。対比を表す表現は一度だけ使う。

whitening		veneers
1. method		1. method
2. invasiveness	⇒	2. invasiveness
3. cost	on the other hand	3. cost
4. duration		4. duration

V. Classification―分類してみよう！
（Lesson 14 ～ 16）

Classification とは同じ性質の物をグループ分けしながら説明する方法である。ポイントはグループ分けをする時の基準（分類の基準）を明確にすることである。例えば野菜を分類する場合、食用部位（分類の基準）によって３つのグループに分けることができる。それらは、fruits（果菜類）, leaves（葉菜類）, roots（根菜類）である。次にそれぞれのグループの特徴と具体例を述べる。果菜類は果実を食べる野菜でトマト、ナス、キュウリなどがある。葉菜類は葉や茎を食べる野菜でキャベツ、アスパラガス、ほうれん草などがある。根菜類は根の部分を食べる野菜でジャガイモ、ニンジン、大根などがある。

同じ野菜の分類でもおいしさなど主観的な基準にすると内容はがらりと変わる。例えば調理法別に分類すると揚げる、煮る、炒める、生、蒸す、茹でる、、、などに分かれる。揚げるとおいしい野菜にはナス、ジャガイモ、玉ねぎなどがある。しかし、おいしさは主観的な尺度であるため分類の仕方は人によって異なる。ここに分類の面白さがある。分類しながらもその人の意見や趣向などが間接的にわかる。

歯科では、臨床科、咬合、カリエスの分類などが考えられる。いずれの分類も客観的な基準で行われる。しかし、上記の野菜のおいしさによる分類のように、自分独自の切り口で分類することもできる。

STEP 1　必要な単語の確認

次の語を英語に直しなさい。括弧が与えられている場合は、そのアルファベットから始めること。

1．〜に分類できる（c、4語で）

2．グループ

3．タイプ

4．〜にしたがって（a、2語で）

5．分類（c）

6．段階（s）

7．〜にしたがって（d、2語で）

8．〜に基づいて（o、4語で）

9．種類（k）

STEP 2　英語で書いてみよう！

1．血液型は4つに分類できる。

2．建物は利用法に基づいて3つに分類できる。

3．ワインはその砂糖含有率（their sugar content）にしたがって分類できる。

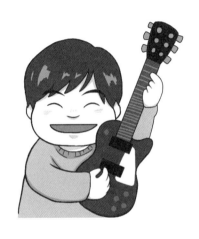

Lesson 14
Classification of clinical departments

Lesson 14. 臨床科の分類

Classification of clinical departments

Message from Dr. Andy

Can you say all the dental departments in English? What if you are at a dental hospital and a foreign patient asks you on which floor is orthodontics? You may also need to know it for the National Board Examination.

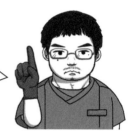

STEP 1 必要な単語の確認

次の各科の名称を日本語で書きなさい。

1. clinics
2. classify
3. Prosthodontics

4. involve / include
5. placement
6. prosthesis

7. denture
8. restoration
9. fillings

10. root canal treatment
11. procedures
12. Oral surgery

13. tooth extraction
14. Orthodontics
15. correction

16. tooth alignment
17. according to

Lesson 14
Classification of clinical departments

STEP 2　英語で書いてみよう！

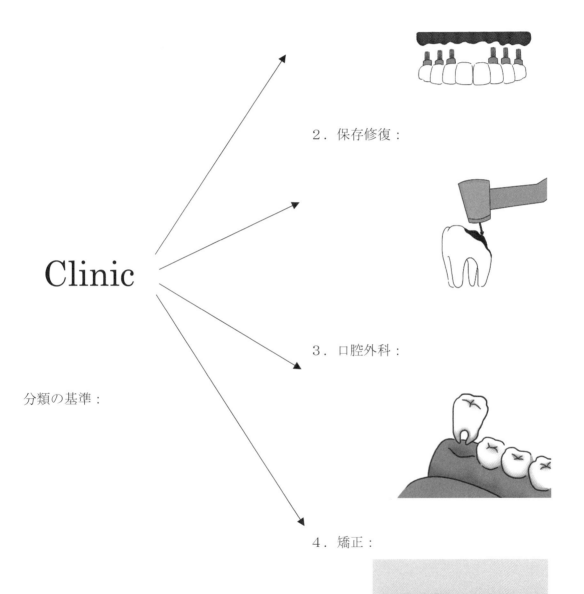

1．補綴：

2．保存修復：

Clinic

3．口腔外科：

分類の基準：

4．矯正：

Lesson 14
Classification of clinical departments

STEP 3　アウトラインを作成する

OUTLINE

Thesis statement（主題）　「臨床科は治療内容別に4つに分類することができる。」

Body（本文）

1.

（補綴：インプラント、ブリッジ、入れ歯などの補綴物の設置などが関連する）

2.

（保存修復：詰物、根管治療、歯周病治療を含む）

3.

（口腔外科：抜歯などの処置が含まれる）

4.

（矯正：歯並びの矯正などの治療を含む）

Conclusion（結論）　「臨床科は治療内容別に補綴、保存修復、口腔外科、矯正に分類することができる。」

アウトラインをもとにエッセイを書いたら、QRコードを読み取って一休み

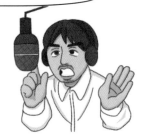

Lesson 14
Classification of clinical departments

STEP 4 英語で言ってみよう！

1. モデルエッセイでシャドーイングをしなさい。
2. 現場での使われ方を **Dialog** で確認しよう。

Dialog

Andy: We need to extract your molar.

Patient: Which tooth will that be?

Andy: Your molar in the lower left jaw.

Patient: Will it hurt?

Andy: Don't worry, I will refer you to the dental hospital. They do a great job.

Patient: A dental hospital! Which department do I go to?

モデルエッセイ： **Classification of clinical departments**

Patient: I see. So, I will be referred to oral surgery.

Andy: Correct.

Patient: When can you resume my orthodontic treatment?

Andy: I would say in about a month or two.

Try this in English 応用編　アウトラインを作成して英語でプレゼンしよう。

タイトル　Classification of shoes　　分類の基準　purpose

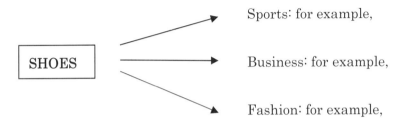

75

Lesson 15
Classification of occlusion

Lesson 15. アングルの咬合の分類

Angle's classification of occlusion

Message from Dr. Andy

Quite a few people suffer from malocclusion. It can be the cause of much discomfort for the patient such as difficulty of pronunciation or chewing. In such cases, I recommend orthodontic treatment to my patients.

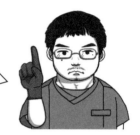

STEP 1　必要な単語の確認

次の語を和訳してみよう。

1. occlusion
2. relation
3. classification

4. overbite
5. upper teeth
6. project

7. further forward
8. lower teeth
9. underbite

Lesson 15
Classification of occlusion

STEP 2　英語で書いてみよう！

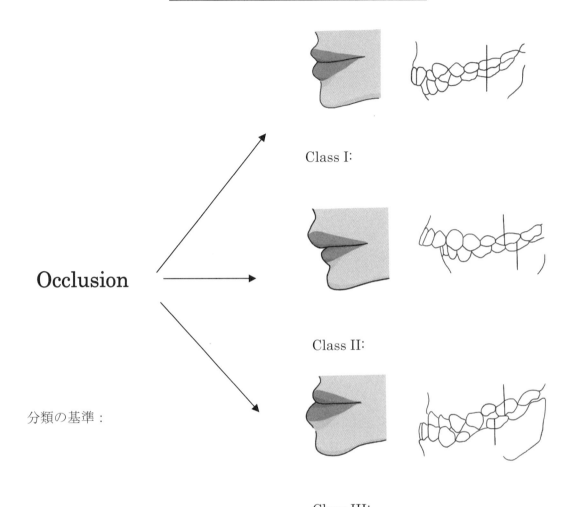

Occlusion

Class I:

Class II:

分類の基準：

Class III:

注：より詳細な分類は以下の通りとなる。

Class I　上顎と下顎の第一大臼歯がずれていない

Class II　下顎第一大臼歯が上顎第一大臼歯に対して後方にある

Class III　下顎第一大臼歯が上顎第一大臼歯に対して前方にある

Lesson 15
Classification of occlusion

STEP 3　アウトラインを作成する

OUTLINE

Thesis statement（主題）「咬合は歯と顎の関係をもとに3つに分類することができる。」

Body（本文）

1.

（このグループでは歯と顎の関係は普通である）

2.

（このグループでは上顎の前歯と上顎は下に対してより前方に出ている）

3.

（このグループでは下顎の前歯と下顎は上に対してより前方に出ている）

Conclusion（結論）「咬合は歯と顎の関係をもとに3つに分類することができる。」

アウトラインをもとにエッセイを書いたら、QRコードを読み取って一休み

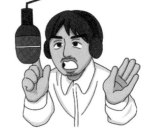

Lesson 15
Classification of occlusion

> STEP 4　英語で言ってみよう！

1．モデルエッセイでシャドーイングをしなさい。
2．現場での使われ方を **Dialog** で確認しよう。

Dialog

Patient: I sometimes have problems pronouncing certain words.

Andy: It may be caused by occlusion problems.

Patient: I always considered my bite as normal.

Andy: Let's see . . . bite down.

Patient: So, how is it?

モデルエッセイ：　Angle's classification of occlusion

Andy: I would say you have a slight overbite. We can do something about it.

Patient: What would that be.

Andy: Orthodontic treatment.

Patient: Oh no! Those metal brackets?

Andy: Not anymore. (showing him a sample)

Try this in English 応用編　アウトラインを作成して英語でプレゼンしよう。

タイトル　Classification of vegetables　　分類の基準　seasons

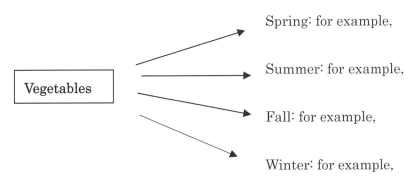

Lesson 16. う蝕の分類

Classification of tooth decay

Message from Dr. Andy

One of the very first steps in becoming a dentist is learning how to classify the different stages of cavities. Be sure to study your textbooks and carefully observe when you go to the hospital for clinics.

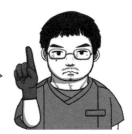

STEP 1　必要な単語の確認

次の語を和訳してみよう。

1. tooth decay
2. according to
3. progression

4. be about to
5. enamel
6. advance to

7. pulp
8. affected
9. roots

10. remain
11. be divided into
12. depend on

Lesson 16
Classification of caries

STEP 2　英語で書いてみよう！

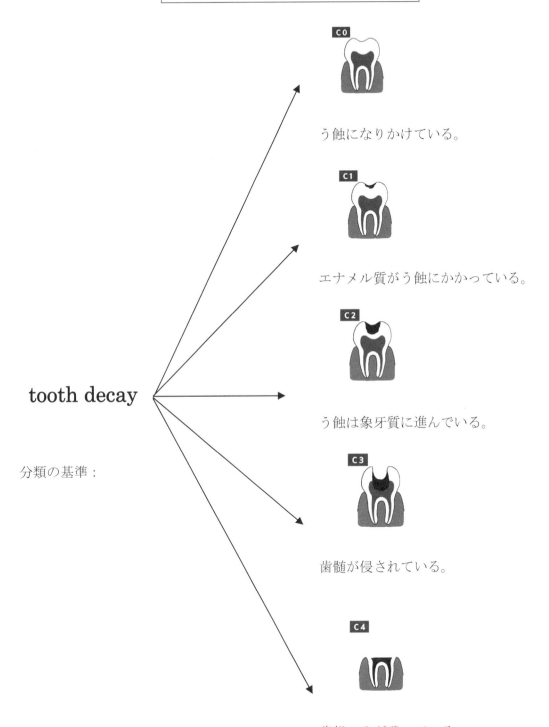

Lesson 16
Classification of caries

STEP 3　アウトラインを作成する

OUTLINE

Thesis statement（主題）「う蝕は進み具合によって5つのステージに分類できる。」

Body（本文）

1.
　（このステージではう蝕がはじまりかけている）
2.
　（このステージではエナメル質がう蝕にかかっている）
3.
　（このステージではう蝕は象牙質に進んでいる）
4.
　（このステージでは歯髄が侵されている）
5.
　（このステージでは歯根のみが残っている）

Conclusion（結論）「う蝕は進み具合によって5つのステージに分類できる。」

アウトラインをもとにエッセイを書いたら、QRコードを読み取って一休み

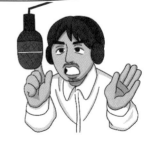

Lesson 16
Classification of caries

STEP 4　英語で言ってみよう！

1．モデルエッセイでシャドーイングをしなさい。
2．現場での使われ方を **Dialog** で確認しよう。

Dialog

(Dr. Andy is doing a checkup on Sally. His assistant is writing down the details on a chart.)

Patient: Hey Dr. Andy, I do not understand Japanese but I think I am hearing a lot of "c-something."

Andy: I was about to explain the results to you just now.

Patient: What does it mean?

本文：**Classification of tooth decay**

Patient: So does it mean that I have several cavities?

Andy: Unfortunately yes.

Patient: Oh my!

Andy: Don't worry. Since they are still in early stages, we can stop further progression.

Patient: Great. What are we waiting for?

Try this in English 応用編　アウトラインを作成して英語でプレゼンしよう。

タイトル（自由に）Classification of ~　　　分類の基準（自由に）

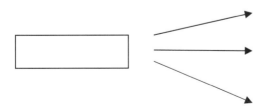

Outline for presentation 01

How to go from the station to the dental clinic

Thesis statement

Body

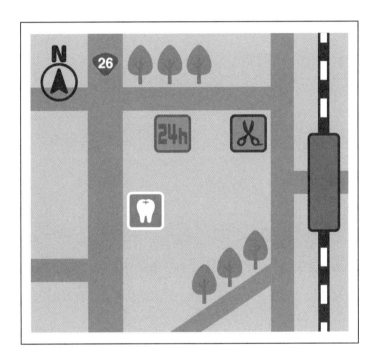

Conclusion
 (Reworded thesis statement)

番号   名前   Score:

Outline for presentation 02

How to brush your teeth

Thesis statement

Body

    1. Choose / bristles

    2. Hold / grip

    3. Apply / 90 / strokes

    4. Apply / 45 / strokes

    5. Brush / surface

    6. Tilt / vertically

Conclusion
    (Reworded thesis statement)

番号   名前   Score:

Outline for presentation 03

How to treat cavities

Thesis statement

Body

   1. Apply

   2. Drill

   3. Fill

   4. Shine

   5. Polish

Conclusion
   (Reworded thesis statement)

番号　　　　　名前　　　　　　　　　　　　　Score:

Outline for presentation 04

The causes of tooth stains

Thesis statement

Body

   1. Smoking / tar and nicotine

   2. Food / pigments

   3. Drinks / tannin

   4. Dead tooth / pulp

Conclusion
   (Reworded thesis statement)

番号　　　　　名前　　　　　　　　　　　Score:

Outline for presentation 05

The causes of bad breath

Thesis statement

Body

  1. Food / strong smelling

  2. Poor oral care / insufficient

  3. Oral diseases / cavities

Conclusion
    (Reworded thesis statement)

番号　　　　　名前　　　　　　　　　　　　Score:

Outline for presentation 06

The causes of stomatitis

Thesis statement

Body

    1. Lack of sleep

    2. External trauma

    3. Unbalanced / vitamin B

Conclusion
    (Reworded thesis statement)

番号　　　　　名前　　　　　　　　　　　Score:

Outline for presentation 07

The effects of poor tooth brushing

Thesis statement

Body

   1. Tooth stains

   2. Tooth decay

   3. Gum trouble

   4. Tooth loss

Conclusion
   (Reworded thesis statement)

番号　　　　　名前　　　　　　　　　　Score:

Outline for presentation 08

Definition of a beautiful smile

Thesis statement

Body

    1. Teeth alignment

    2. Teeth color

    3. Facial expressions

Conclusion
    (Reworded thesis statement)

番号   名前   Score:

Outline for presentation 09

Definition of a good dentist

Thesis statement

Body

   1. Communication skills

   2. Respect

   3. Knowledge

   4. Treatment skills

Conclusion
   (Reworded thesis statement)

番号　　　　名前　　　　　　　　　　　Score:

Outline for presentation 10

The difference between dental schools

Thesis statement

Body

  1. Graduates / Australia / Japan

  2. Years / Australia / Japan

  3. Clinics / Australia / Japan

  4. Licensed / Australia / Japan

Conclusion
   (Reworded thesis statement)

番号   名前   Score:

Outline for presentation 11

The difference between metal crowns and ceramic crowns

Thesis statement

Body

   1. Insurance / metal / ceramic

   2. Appearance / metal / ceramic

   3. Durable / metal / ceramic

   4. Allergy / metal / ceramic

Conclusion
   (Reworded thesis statement)

番号　　　　　名前　　　　　　　　　　　Score:

Outline for presentation 12

The difference between implants and bridges

Thesis statement

Body

  1. Strain / implants / bridges

  2. Maintenance / implants / bridges

  3. Time / implants / bridges

  4. Cost / implants / bridges

Conclusion
   (Reworded thesis statement)

番号　　　　名前　　　　　　　　　　　Score:

Outline for presentation 13

The difference between whitening and veneers

Thesis statement

Body

   1. Conducted by / whitening / veneers

   2. Invasive / whitening / veneers

   3. Cost / whitening / veneers

   4. Effect / whitening / veneers

Conclusion
   (Reworded thesis statement)

番号　　　　　名前　　　　　　　　　　　Score:

Outline for presentation 14

Classification of clinical departments

Thesis statement

Body

   1. Prosthodontics / placement

   2. Restoration / fillings

   3. Oral surgery / extractions

   4. Orthodontics / alignment

Conclusion
   (Reworded thesis statement)

番号   名前   Score:

Outline for presentation 15

Angle's classification of occlusion

Thesis statement

Body

   1. Class I / normal

   2. Class II / overbite / project forward

   3. Class III / underbite / project forward

Conclusion
   (Reworded thesis statement)

番号   名前   Score:

Outline for presentation 16

Classification of tooth decay

Thesis statement

Body

    1. C0 / start

    2. C1 / enamel

    3. C2 / dentin

    4. C3 / pulp

    5. C4 / roots

Conclusion
    (Reworded thesis statement)

番号   名前   Score:

著者紹介

藤田淳一（ふじた　じゅんいち）　大阪歯科大学英語教室

岡隼人（おか　はやと）　大阪歯科大学英語教室

安東大器（あんどう　たいき）安東第二歯科医院

岡村友玄（おかむら　ともはる）　大阪歯科大学口腔病理学講座

吉川美弘（よしかわ　よしひろ）　大阪歯科大学生化学講座

Illustrations by noriko
Cover artwork by たろう

Special thanks to
Julia Gadd, William Hall, Dr. Mutti, Dr. Hideyuki Okamura and Keita Kawamura

DjD の動画をもっと見たい人はこちらへ

YouTube
チャンネル登録も是非お願いします。

QRコードシリーズ
動画でわかる歯科英語
― 16レッスンで鍛える表現力 ―

発　行　日	2019年4月1日　初版第1刷発行	
著　　　者	藤田淳一／岡　隼人／安東大器	
	岡村友玄／吉川美弘	
発　行　者	杉田宗詞	
発　行　所	図書出版　浪速社	
	〒540-0037　大阪市中央区内平野町2－2－7－502	
	TEL 06（6942）5032　FAX 06（6943）1346	
印刷・製本	株式会社ディーネット	

―禁無断転載―

2019年 © 藤田淳一／岡　隼人／安東大器／岡村友玄／吉川美弘

乱丁落丁はお取り替えいたします
ISBN978-4-88854-521-1